"With amazing clarity, Dr. Jennings cuts through the many divergent God constructs to expose the powerful impact these differing views have upon our brains and bodies. Not everything taught about God is healthy—read this book and learn how your belief about God is changing you."

Gregory L. Jantz, Ph.D., C.E.D.S., founder, The Center, Inc.

"It has been said that our thoughts reflect who we are (Proverbs 23:7). Dr. Jennings challenges us with a synthesis of neurobiology and theology that elaborates on this concept."

Michael Lyles, M.D., Lyles and Crawford Clinical Consulting

"Dr. Tim Jennings has asked the troublesome questions about God's character and answered them in a simple and compelling way that clears away the lies about him so that you find yourself falling deeper in love with him. It's a must-read for every inquiring mind. Once you understand the physiology of the brain and how it responds to love versus selfishness, as explained by Dr. Jennings, you will realize that the choice for love is the only one that will renew the mind and result in good mental health."

Kay Kuzma, Ed.D., president of Family Matters Ministry

"Paying attention to the findings of neuroscience is tantamount to paying attention to God's creation. And doing that leads us—with the proper guide—to God's story and his intentions for us. Tim Jennings is that proper guide. An experienced healer with a palpable spirit of humility, he takes the reader past the trite, superficial motifs of easy spirituality that clutter our emotional landscapes and grounds you first in the nature of the God of Scripture. He then further explores that in which God grounded the first humans—the body, and namely, the brain. With compelling stories of challenge and transformation, Dr. Jennings deftly weaves together a deeply thoughtful theology of the living Word with the complex nature of the organ that our heart calls home. Read this book to know God more fully. Read this book to know your brain more fully. And see how knowing God will change your brain—and your life—in ways you never thought possible."

Curt Thompson, M.D., psychiatrist and author of *The Soul of Shame*

"What makes this book truly remarkable is the artful way Dr. Jennings combines the latest understanding in brain physiology with practical and compelling real-life stories. Although this book is easy to understand for the layperson, the implications Dr. Jennings makes about the design of the human brain, how it can be damaged and how it can be healed are profound. I don't know of another book that so beautifully describes how our mind can be restored back to the way God originally designed it to be."

Brad Cole, M.D., director of neuroscience education,
Loma Linda University School of Medicine

"If you are ready to take your relationship with God to the next level, if you are ready to move closer to the source of all truth, if you are ready for an evidence-based approach to knowing God, this book is for you. Dr. Jennings's patient cases and illustrations make complex ideas simple and easy to understand as he powerfully documents, through brain science, how our beliefs about God change us."

Tim Clinton, president, American Association of Christian Counselors

EXPANDED EDITION

THE G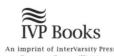D-SHAPED BRAIN

How Changing Your View of God
Transforms Your Life

Timothy R. Jennings, M.D.

≈≈
IVP Books
An imprint of InterVarsity Press
Downers Grove, Illinois

InterVarsity Press
P.O. Box 1400, Downers Grove, IL 60515-1426
ivpress.com
email@ivpress.com

Second edition ©2017 by Timothy R. Jennings
First edition ©2013 by Timothy R. Jennings

InterVarsity Press® is the book-publishing division of InterVarsity Christian Fellowship/USA®, a movement of students and faculty active on campus at hundreds of universities, colleges and schools of nursing in the United States of America, and a member movement of the International Fellowship of Evangelical Students. For information about local and regional activities, visit intervarsity.org.

All Scripture quotations, unless otherwise indicated, are taken from THE HOLY BIBLE, NEW INTERNATIONAL VERSION®, NIV® Copyright © 1973, 1978, 1984, 2011 by Biblica, Inc.™ Used by permission. All rights reserved worldwide.

Image of the human brain on p. 7 used with permission from Simon Harrison.

While any stories in this book are true, some names and identifying information in this book may have been changed to protect the privacy of the individuals involved.

Published in association with the literary agency of D. C. Jacobson & Associates, Lake Oswego, Oregon. www.dcjacobson.com.

Cover Design: Cindy Kiple
Interior Design: Beth McGill
Images: Head with gear inside: CSA Images/Color Printstock Collection/Getty Images
        Atom: Yulia Glam/iStockphoto

ISBN 978-0-8308-4495-1 (print)
ISBN 978-0-8308-9235-8 (digital)

Printed in the United States of America ∞

Library of Congress Cataloging-in-Publication Data

Jennings, Timothy R., 1961-
    The God-shaped brain : how changing your view of God transforms your life / Timothy R. Jennings.
      pages cm
    Includes bibliographical references and index.
    ISBN 978-0-8308-3416-7 (pbk. : alk. paper)
      1. God (Christianity) 2. Thought and thinking—Religious aspects—Christianity. 3. Christian life. 4. Mental health—Religious aspects—Christianity. I. Title.
    BT103.J46 2013
    231—dc23

                                                          2013001332

P   18   17   16   15   14   13   12   11   10   9   8   7   6   5   4   3   2
Y   32   31   30   29   28   27   26   25   24   23   22   21   20   19   18

Contents

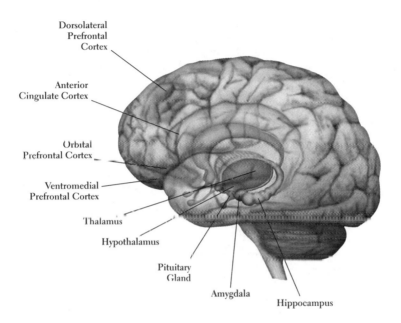

Dorsolateral
Prefrontal
Cortex

Anterior
Cingulate Cortex

Orbital
Prefrontal Cortex

Ventromedial
Prefrontal Cortex

Thalamus

Hypothalamus

Pituitary
Gland

Amygdala

Hippocampus

Diagram of the human brain

Preface

The thing always happens that you really believe in;
and the belief in a thing makes it happen.

FRANK LLOYD WRIGHT

RECENTLY, MY ELEVEN-YEAR-OLD NEPHEW and fourteen-year-old niece, who have not been raised in a churchgoing family, attended church. The sermon was a discourse on God's wrath and was delivered with a fiery intensity designed to "shock and awe." After this searing exhortation, both came home distraught and reported that the preacher presented a god that scared them—one that, if true, they would never want to believe in.

I wondered, *Would Jesus be happy if we presented him in such a way that the children would not want to be with him or know him?* Isn't something wrong if in talking about God we frighten the children? Do we help or hurt, heal or injure, when we present a God that incites fear? Does it even matter whether our view of God is good, bad or ugly? It *does* matter, more than we ever realized—to the point of changing our brain structure! Although we have power over what we believe, what we believe holds real power over us—power to heal and power to destroy.

Late one night in a small Alabama cemetery, Vance Vanders had a run-in with the local witch doctor, who wafted a bottle of unpleasant-smelling liquid in front of his face, and told him he was about to die and that no one could save him.

Back home, Vanders took to his bed and began to deteri-
orate. Some weeks later, emaciated and near death, he was admitted to the local hospital, where doctors were unable to find
a cause for his symptoms or slow his decline. Only then did his
wife tell one of the doctors, Drayton Doherty, of the hex.

Doherty thought long and hard. The next morning, he
called Vanders's family to his bedside. He told them that the
previous night he had lured the witch doctor back to the cemetery, where he had choked him against a tree until he explained how the curse worked. The medicine man had, he
said, rubbed lizard eggs into Vanders's stomach, which had
hatched inside his body. One reptile remained, which was
eating Vanders from the inside out.

Doherty then summoned a nurse who had, by prior ar-
rangement, filled a large syringe with a powerful emetic [a substance which induces vomiting]. With great ceremony, he in-
spected the instrument and injected its contents into Vanders's
arm. A few minutes later, Vanders began to gag and vomit uncontrollably. In the midst of it all, unnoticed by everyone in the
room, Doherty produced his pièce de résistance—a green
lizard he had stashed in his black bag. "Look what has come
out of you Vance," he cried. "The voodoo curse is lifted."

Vanders did a double take, lurched backwards to the head of
the bed, then drifted into a deep sleep. When he woke the next
day he was alert and ravenous. He quickly regained his strength
and was discharged a week later.[1]

Vance is not alone. Medical literature is replete with case reports
of patients dying, not from actual illness, but from *believing* they
were sick, from the *fear* they were going to die. Surgeons routinely
avoid operating on patients who are convinced they will die during
surgery. The risk is too great.[2]

In the 1970s, Sam Shoeman was diagnosed with liver cancer and told he had only months to live. A few months after his death, the autopsy revealed the doctors were wrong. He had only one small tumor still contained within the liver—not a life-threatening stage of cancer. Sam Shoeman did not die from liver cancer; he died from *believing* he was dying of liver cancer. Our beliefs change us mentally, physically and spiritually.[3]

Our brains are constantly in a state of flux. Moment by moment new neurons are developing and new circuits are being laid down, new axons and dendrites are forming for the facilitating of new messages to the neurons. At the same time, unused connections are removed, dormant nerve tracks are pruned back and unused neurons are deleted. Incredibly, our beliefs, thoughts, behaviors and even our diets change our brain structure, ultimately changing who we are.

Throughout this book we will explore the amazing ability of our brains to adapt, change and rewire based on the choices we make, the beliefs we hold and the God we worship—as different "God-concepts" affect the brain differently. My goal with this book is to reveal God in the clearest way possible, to demonstrate how our belief in God changes us and to display his methods on a practical level. I also offer a new methodology in the study of God, which I have termed the Integrative Evidence-Based Approach, which incorporates and requires harmony of three threads, Scripture (with special emphasis on the life of Jesus), God's laws in science and nature, and our experience—all studied with a humble mind under the guidance of the Holy Spirit.

In their book *Rediscovering the Scandal of the Cross*, Joel Green and Mark Baker observe that our views of God are influenced by the social environment of the times. Then they ask a most pertinent question: "Which of our affirmations [about God] are true? and, Who decides?"[4] I suggest that God has provided testable evidence that, if incorporated into our decision making, enable us to determine which are true and which are not. If we study science without Scripture, we risk falling into the ditch of atheistic evolutionism; on the other hand, the study of Scripture separated from God's laws in nature risks theologies that misrepresent God and distort his character.

To maintain a healthy balance, we must use the Bible and harmonize it with science and our experience to separate the various views of God, demonstrating the marked difference each view has on our mental, physical and relational health. In this book I will explore how a change in one's thinking about God and Scripture results in the healing of mind, body and relationships, while holding to distorted God-concepts bring pain, suffering and, ultimately, death.

I am a psychiatrist. I am not a seminary-trained theologian. My approach is likely to be very different from that of a seminary professor, and for good reason. The Bible says we are in a battle, with weapons that demolish arguments and pretensions that are opposed to God, and our thoughts are to be harmonized with Christ.

The battlefield on which the war between Christ and Satan is fought is the mind. As a practicing Christian psychiatrist, I routinely engage in spiritual warfare—thus in this book I approach the interpretation of Scripture as a physician, a mind specialist and a seasoned "battlefield" veteran. While Scripture was written by diverse authors over many generations, usually for a specific audience and with a contextual application, it was also inspired by the same Holy Spirit and, as such, presents an overriding theme, a central thread centering on God's character of love. I take the position that it is not only legitimate but also vitally necessary to take Scripture as a whole, tying together all the various pieces to obtain the fullest revelation of God's character.

Therefore, I accept interpretations that harmonize with Scripture as a whole (especially the truth about God as revealed in Christ), and with God's testable laws and that bring healing (our objective life experience). But you will see that I consider and reject interpretations that are inconsistent with Scripture as a whole (contradict the evidence Christ provided), violate God's testable laws, or are destructive to physical and mental health. I encourage you to be scientific, be critical, examine everything I say—do not merely accept my claims but compare my findings with the evidence of Scripture and science. Test the ideas put forth and come to your own conclusions.

Finally, as you read this book you will be reminded of a foundational principle of the Reformation—the priesthood of believers, the reality that God has created each one of us in his image, each with our own brain, to be a temple where God dwells by his Spirit. As such, all believers, in union with God, are capable of discerning Scripture correctly without the need of a priest or theologian to do their thinking for them. Naturally this does not mean we cannot benefit from the insights, expertise and experience of pastors or theology professors, but rather, we must not surrender our thinking to other human beings. Again, I invite you to examine the evidence and, "Do not conform any longer to the pattern of this world, but be transformed by the renewing of your mind. Then you will be able to test and approve what God's will is—his good, pleasing and perfect will" (Rom 12:2).

Acknowledgments

To MY PATIENTS, THANK YOU for the privilege of being your doctor. Your growth, your healing, your transformed lives have filled my life with joy. Thank you!

To Christie, thank you for your patience, encouragement and support.

To Simon Harrison, thank you for sharing your artistic talents and providing the diagram of the brain.

To all my friends who have kept me in prayer, thank you, may this book be a blessing to you.

All patient accounts described in this book are true. All names and identifying information have been changed to protect confidentiality. Some of the cases presented include information from multiple persons to further protect confidentiality. The cases presented in this book are selected to demonstrate problems that can arise when distorted views of God are held, and how a change in God-constructs can bring healing. However, not all patients have problems with their concepts of God, and changing a God-concept will not resolve all mental health problems. Many people suffer from illnesses that attack the physical brain, such as Alzheimer's, schizophrenia, bipolar disorder and autism, and changing one's God-concept will not resolve these disorders. Nevertheless it will be demonstrated that distorted God-concepts, while not directly causative of many disorders, are unhealthy, and holding to them will undermine health and healing.

God, the Brain and What Went Wrong

God Is Love

Love is life. All, everything that I understand,
I understand only because I love.
Everything is, everything exists, only because I love.
Everything is united by it alone.

LEO TOLSTOY

"DON'T CRY," I said gently.

But she was crying uncontrollably, her body shaking with each sob, and the tears flooded down her cheeks until they cascaded onto her blouse, forming what looked like little dark pools.

I waited, and eventually she began to speak, just snippets at first. A word, gasp, sob, another word. But slowly she disclosed what was tormenting her.

"It's all my fault!" More tears.

"What's your fault?"

"I can't have children. Oh, God!"

"Why do you say it's your fault?"

More sobs, and with her face buried in her hands, she told me that when she was a teenager she had gotten pregnant and had an abortion. The abortion was routine, no complications, no injuries, so I wondered why she couldn't have children.

Then she said, "I can't have children because God is punishing me. My pastor told me that I murdered my child and as punishment God won't ever let me have children."

As I sat listening to my patient cry, empathizing, I considered what her core problem was. Did her despair primarily stem from the fact that she had fertility problems, or from her belief about God and the perception of being punished? Could her central psychological stress be arising not from her objective reproductive condition but rather a distorted view of God? Does it make a difference to one's health to believe, as some had suggested, that God was punishing her for mistakes she had made? Would it be helpful, even healing, if she came to believe that, rather than punishing her, God was crying with her?

Have you ever been hurt and wondered, *Where is God, what is he doing, why didn't he intervene?* Or worse, have you ever thought God was punishing you or someone you knew?

Have you ever been frustrated with, confused by or wrestled with conflicting views about God? Were you ever taught that God is love, but that he also punishes and inflicts pain for disobedience—not to redeem and discipline but to torture and destroy? Have you battled with fear of God? Have you considered the possibility that your view of God could be affecting your mental, physical and relational health?

During my life I've had many questions about God and how our beliefs about him affect us. I have seen countless lives changed, for good or ill, based on a turn in a belief about God. And I have spent more than two decades searching for answers in Scripture and science for truth about God that heals and restores. I hope some of the answers I have found will be beneficial to you.

A TIME BEFORE HUMANITY

As a believer in God, I realized that the most reasonable place to start my search for God-concepts that heal was in the beginning. So I used the Bible and my imagination to travel back in time. I journeyed past the point I was born, past the origin of my parents, grandparents and great-great-great-grandparents, even sailing beyond Adam and Eve to a time when only God and the angels existed. The Bible tells us in Job 38:7 that the angels shouted for joy at the creation of the earth. According to Scripture, there was a time before any human being existed.

At long last I arrived at a time when the universe was free from all defect—a perfect place. Then carefully, prayerfully, I went even further, all the way back before the angels, to a point when there was only God, the eternal triune love. "In the beginning was the Word, and the Word was with God, and the Word was God. He was with God in the beginning" (Jn 1:1-2).

In my imagination I wondered what the universe was like then. But I quickly realized it was beyond my comprehension, so I retraced my steps, returning in time, and saw the universe spring forth from the mind of God. Flashes of light, explosions of color, of suns, planets, galaxies forming, taking shape. "Through him [Jesus] all things were made; without him nothing was made that has been made." "For in him all things were created: things in heaven and on earth, visible and invisible, whether thrones or powers or rulers or authorities; all things have been created through him and for him" (Jn 1:3; Col 1:16).

After observing the creation of inanimate nature, my imagination saw Love's true aim: life. Life burst forth from the heart of God; beautiful, radiant and pure. Like Michelangelo's careful brushstrokes, Handel's lofty choruses and Shakespeare's masterful sonnets, angelic beings sprang forth from the love of God. I saw Jesus turn to his Father and say: "Look, Father, aren't they wonderful?" And the Father responded, "Yes, Son, they're perfect! Let's make some more beautiful creatures; free, intelligent and capable of genuine love." And soon the heavens were filled with the sound of rejoicing, laughter, singing and happiness.

In awe I realized that God himself is the great source of all life. Then it struck me. If God is the originator of all creation, then he is the wellspring that the parameters, blueprints and foundational designs for life arise. God's very nature, essence and being is the source code of life, health and happiness, the template on which life is built! He designed and constructed life to operate only in harmony with his own character, because it is from him that all things hold together: "He [Christ] is before all things, and in him all things hold together" (Col 1:17).

GOD—THE TEMPLATE FOR LIFE

The implications of this concept were staggering. Humanity was patterned after God. Therefore, the critical issue I had to understand, in order to understand God's original design for humanity and the functioning of the human brain, was *God himself*. I needed to know the essential, core, defining characteristic of God—who he is. Is he good, or as my niece and nephew heard at church, hostile and mean? I turned to Scripture and then to nature, holding to only that which was found evidenced in both, and what I discovered changed my life.

The core, central, primary characteristic of God . . . is love (1 Jn 4:8). Not the silly, finite, flimsy, emotional, wax-fruit imposter we sometimes call love, but a boundless, eternal, bottomless, never-ending, reality of goodness on which the cosmos is built! A love that lasts, that creates, that is constant.

God is love. The Bible does not say God *is* forgiveness, even though he is forgiving; or that God *is* knowledge, even though he is all-knowing; or that God *is* power, even though he is all-powerful. All other attributes are, like facets on a diamond, radiant windows into the heart of God. But with regard to love, God does not merely act it out—he embodies it!

This all-encompassing love is alien to our world, foreign to sinful earth and is described by the Bible in shockingly counterearthly language, "[love] is not self-seeking" (1 Cor 13:5). Love does not trample others on "Black Friday" to get the best after-Thanksgiving deal. Love does not treat your coworker with disrespect. Love is not found after six beers with a stranger in a Friday night bar.

Love doesn't seek self; it seeks others. Love's heart burns for others. Love is outward moving, giving and beneficial to others. Love sacrifices self for the good of others. Because God is love, his very essence, nature and character is outward moving, other-centered, giving and beneficial to others. "For God loved the world so much that he *gave* his only Son." "The greatest love you can have for your friends is to *give* your life for them." "This is how we know what love is: Christ *gave* his life for us. We too, then, ought to give our lives for others!" (Jn 3:16; 15:13; 1 Jn 3:16 CNT, emphasis mine). God's very nature is other-centered love. We know that love "burns like blazing fire, like a mighty flame. Many waters cannot quench love; rivers cannot sweep it away" (Song 8:6-7). And this passionate, selfless, blazing love radiates from God like energy from the sun.

> The Ancient of Days took his seat.
> His clothing was as white as snow;
>   the hair of his head was white like wool.
> His throne was flaming with fire,
>   and its wheels were all ablaze.
> A river of fire was flowing,
>   coming out from before him.
> Thousands upon thousands attended him;
>   ten thousand times ten thousand stood before him.
>   (Dan 7:9-10)

As I continued my search, Romans 1:20 suddenly exploded with new meaning: "For since the creation of the world God's invisible qualities—his eternal power and *divine nature*—have been clearly seen, being understood from *what has been made*, so that people are without excuse" (emphasis mine). God's nature of love is seen in creation because all nature, all life, is built, designed, constructed to operate on the template of God's love.

God's law of love is the outward flow of his personhood in the constant dispersion of himself to create, uphold and sustain the universe. This giving, outward-moving, other-centered love is the design on which all creation was constructed to operate. The law of love is the principle of selfless giving, which is the foundation upon which all life is built to function. Simply put, the law of love is the law of life! Harmony with this principle brings life, health and happiness. Disharmony, naturally, results in pain, suffering and death. "We know that we have passed from death to life, because we love each other. Anyone who does not love remains in death" (1 Jn 3:14).

Suddenly, as this concept sank deep into my mind, the world had new meaning. Love flowing from God was transforming my heart. My eyes were opening, and I saw the law of love everywhere I looked.

LOVE IN NATURE

The oceans *give* their waters to the clouds, which rain over the land, *giving* their waters to form the lakes, rivers and streams, which in turn *give* their waters to the plants and animals, ultimately *giving* back to the oceans to start the circle again. The law of love is the circle of giving that is the law of life. All life is built on this principle because all life originates with God. If a body of water separates from the circle and ceases to flow, it stagnates and everything in it dies. God gave us a powerful illustration in the body of water called the Dead Sea. The Dead Sea takes from the Jordan River but gives nothing in return. What happens in that body of water? The name says it all.

We see the circle of love, the law of life, in everything God creates. In every breath we demonstrate giving: we give away carbon dioxide to the plants, and the plants give back oxygen to us. Imagine if you were to decide, "I don't want to be a part of the circle of giving. If my body makes carbon dioxide, it's mine; I have the right to it. You can't have it." The only way to do that is to stop breathing—to die. If we hoard the product of our breathing, maybe by putting a bag over our heads, the carbon dioxide becomes the poisoning agent that kills us. In all life we see this circle of giving, which is the law of love.

Consider electricity: when electricity moves through metal wires it does so by the movement of electrons from one atom to another. They flow in what we call a current, but they can only do so if the current forms a complete circle, which we call a circuit. When you flip the switch to turn on a light, you have "closed" the electrical circuit, thus forming a complete "circle" allowing the electrons to flow and the light to come on. Conversely, when you flip the switch to turn off the light, you break the circle, and the electrons cannot flow. It is only when the circles (circuits) are complete that electricity flows. This is how nature was built to operate. The law of love is the design template for all God's creation because all life flows from him and God is love.

God has written his law of love—his circle of beneficence—in all of nature because it is the design schematic for life's basic operation. The planets of our solar system *circle* around the sun, and the sun *gives* away its energy freely. Plants receive the sun's energy and, through metabolic "circles" internal to the plants (Calvin-Benson Cycle), convert the sun's energy into chemical energy. The plants give this energy to us in the form of fruits, nuts, grains and vegetables, and in the process give us oxygen to breathe. We receive the food from the plants and, through a series of metabolic "circles" internal to us (citric acid cycle), use the energy and convert the molecules to water, carbon dioxide and byproducts of digestion, which we give back to the earth, to fertilize the plants. It's a never-ending circle of giving.

In every living system, if it is to be healthy, the circle must not be broken. But this principle has implications with even further reach. This is true even in our economy. If the economy is to be

healthy, the money has to be in *circulation*. If you take the money
out of circulation, the economy dies. This happened during the
Great Depression when everyone ran to the bank to withdraw all
they had deposited. President Roosevelt responded with large
government spending programs, pumping currency back into circulation, and the economy revived.

We see the circle of love in everything God created. The planets
circle around the sun. The solar system circles in the galaxy, and the
galaxies circle in the universe. Everything God creates gives freely in
other-centered circles. I don't think it's a coincidence that when the
prophet Ezekiel looked into heaven in a vision, what he saw symbol-
izing the foundation of God's government was a wheel within a
wheel, a rotation within a rotation, a moving circle within a moving
circle (Ezek 10:1-10).

God tried to teach us this basic truth within the Old Testament
sacrificial system. In that system, a sinner would confess his sin on the
head of an animal, and then the sinner would cut the animal's *circulation*. The life is in the blood (Lev 17:11), and it circles throughout the
body. The teaching is amazingly simple: sin severs the circle of life.

The lifeblood of an animal is, naturally, its physical blood. The
lifeblood of the economy is money; of an appliance, electricity. But
the lifeblood of the universe is love, which flows from God through
Christ to all creation and back to God through Christ again. This is
God's design template. This is the blueprint on which humanity was
created to operate!

Whenever the circle of giving—the circle of love—is broken,
pain, suffering and death inevitably follow. And it is only the love
flowing from God that restores life, health and happiness.

NOT EASY TO SEE

As beautiful as God's character of love is, it was not easy for me to
see. It wasn't easy because I had not lived in harmony with God's
love. I had accepted a different version of his love: a common, earthly

version I had learned even at my church. What I learned suggested that love is authoritarian and commanding, that love rules over and inflicts just punishment for disobedience. It was hard for me to realize how twisted this assumption of my heart truly was, and I began to discover that bright light hurts when we are used to the darkness.

In 2006 Baylor University took a national survey to evaluate how people viewed God. They found that only 23 percent of people viewed him as benevolent or loving, while 32 percent saw the Almighty as authoritarian, 16 percent as critical and 24 percent as distant. Five percent claimed to be atheist.[1]

Does it matter which God-concept we hold to? Recent brain research by Dr. Newberg at the University of Pennsylvania has documented that all forms of contemplative meditation were associated with positive brain changes—but the greatest improvements occurred when participants meditated specifically on a God of love. Such meditation was associated with growth in the prefrontal cortex (the part of the brain right behind our forehead where we reason, make judgments and experience Godlike love) and subsequent increased capacity for empathy, sympathy, compassion and altruism. But here's the most astonishing part. Not only does other-centered love increase when we worship a God of love, but sharp thinking and memory improve as well. In other words, worshiping a God of love actually stimulates the brain to heal and grow.[2]

However, when we worship a god other than one of love—a being who is punitive, authoritarian, critical or distant—fear circuits are activated and, if not calmed, will result in chronic inflammation and damage to both brain and body. As we bow before authoritarian gods, our characters are slowly changed to be less like Jesus. Truly, by beholding we are changed, not only in character, but our neural circuitry as well[3] (2 Cor 3:18 KJV).

APPLICATION TO YOUR LIFE TODAY

In this first of several application sections throughout the book, below are actions you can take to apply God's principles to your life in order to experience transformation here and now.

1. Practice examining the three threads of evidence: Scripture, testable laws in nature and your own experience. Can you identify God's character of love from Scripture? Does the evidence provided in the life of Christ confirm God's love as understood in the rest of Scripture? Do you see the principle of love revealed in nature? Identify where in your own life you have experienced self-sacrificial love manifested toward you, and where you have manifested such love toward others. What impact did that love have on you and others?

2. The law of love is an expression of God's character and the template on which life is built. As God never changes so, too, his law of love never changes; this means the law of love is a tool we can use to test various theories about God. The world is filled with numerous religions, denominations and views about God. The law of love is a clarifying standard to filter the various views of God. Any theory that, in effect, has God violating the law of love would be recognized as incorrect.

   This law, then, is a divine boundary line demarcating our theological "safe zone." Require all your interpretations of Scripture to harmonize with this testable law. For instance, the Bible describes God, in certain places, as angry or wrathful. How do you interpret the meaning of those descriptions of God in the Bible as angry? Are your conclusions in harmony with the law of love, or is there conflict? If you struggle with this question, keep reading; later in this book we will explore how God's wrath can be understood to be in harmony with the law of love.

3. Perhaps the most important application of this law is choosing to live in harmony with it. Because the law of love is the law of life, choosing to impart love to others is one of God's methods to strengthen you. "A generous person will be enriched and one who

gives water will get water" (Prov 11:25 NRSV). Harmony with God's design promotes better health, here and now. Just as following the manufacturer's design protocol for your car and using unleaded gas rather than diesel results in more efficient function, so choosing to operate in harmony with God's design for life results in better mental and physical health. And scientific research demonstrates that, in fact, giving is living:

> Dozens of studies over several decades have examined relationships between volunteer work and health-related outcomes. Most studies have shown positive volunteering-health associations. Among youth, evidence suggests that volunteer work is associated with a plethora of positive developmental outcomes, such as academic achievement, civic responsibility, and life skills that include leadership and interpersonal self-confidence (Astin & Sax 1998).[4]

Four studies between 1996 and 2003 evaluated the effect of volunteerism and longevity in the elderly. Controlling for confounding variables, such as health when entering the study, all four studies "reported that volunteers tended to live statistically longer than those who did not volunteer."[5]

Not only do volunteers live longer but they live better too:

> Several studies have examined the relationship between volunteering and physical functioning. Moen, Dempster-McClain, and Williams (1989) studied 427 women who resided in upstate New York and were both wives and mothers in 1956. Over the next 30 years, compared to nonvolunteers, women who did any volunteering had better physical functioning in 1986, after adjusting for baseline health status, level of education, and number of life roles. Similarly, Luoh and Herzog (2002) found that, compared to nonvolunteers or those volunteering less than 100 hours, those who were volunteering 100 hours or more in 1998 were ap-

proximately 30% less likely to experience physical functioning limitations, even after adjusting for demographics, socioeconomic status, baseline functioning limitations, health status, paid employment, exercise, smoking and social connections. Moorow-Howell and colleagues (2003) examined data collected between 1986 and 1994 from more than 1,500 U.S. adults, finding that volunteering predicted significantly less functional disability 3 to 5 years later, after adjusting for demographics, socioeconomic status, marital status, and informal social integration.[6]

Just as the Bible teaches, to give is to live. This is how God designed life to function. So why do so many, including myself, struggle to give? In our next chapter we will explore: (1) why there is so much exploitation, violence and selfishness in the world; (2) what happened to God's original design, the circle of love; and (3) how our view of God makes the critical difference.

2

The Human Brain and Broken Love

Every violation of truth is not only a sort of suicide in the liar,
but is a stab at the health of human society.

RALPH WALDO EMERSON

IN FEBRUARY 2011 HUMAN BRAINPOWER faced off against Watson, IBM's supercomputer, in a battle of knowledge and processing speed on the popular TV show *Jeopardy*. Who would win? Ken Jennings and Brad Rutter, the top two all-time *Jeopardy* winners, or Watson, IBM's synthetic creation? After three intense matches, Watson had defeated the human competition. Watson's win had some fearing that computers had finally advanced beyond the human brain. But, I say, not so fast—let's do a little comparison between Watson and a human brain and see how well the human brain stands up.

Watson is composed of 90 IBM Power 750 servers, each 6.9 inches high, 17.3 inches wide, 28.7 inches deep and weighing 120 pounds, for a total weight of over 10,000 pounds—housed in 10 large racks in a room approximately 12 feet by 10 feet.[1] Watson contains 2,880 Power7 processors, with each processor consisting of 8 cores containing 1.2 billion transistors and 16 terabytes of RAM,[2] processing 500 gigabytes of information per sec (1 million books/sec).[3]

In comparison, the human brain weighs about 3 pounds and is contained within the small space inside the skull. The brain is estimated to have more than 100 billion nerve cells and over one trillion supporting cells. Each nerve cell can have up to 10 thousand connections to other nerve cells, which makes the brain highly interconnected with some estimates of over a quadrillion connections.[4]

The human brain holds approximately 1.25 terabytes of data and performs at approximately 100 teraflops[5] (one hundred trillion point operations per second). Watson holds 1 terabyte of data and performs at 80 teraflops (eighty trillion point operations per second).[6]

In addition to actually having greater speed and storage capacity than Watson, the human brain, being housed in the body, is highly portable and can choose to move itself from place to place; Watson cannot. The human brain can experience emotions; Watson cannot. The human brain can rewire itself based on new experience or a change in understanding; Watson cannot. The human brain can grow new components (neurons); Watson cannot. Ultimately, the human brain turns out to be the most marvelous piece of engineering known, far beyond human ingenuity and immeasurably more complex than Watson.

Then why did Watson win? According to Ken Jennings, it had nothing to do with knowledge or ability to answer the questions. It all came down to who could ring in fastest. Jennings said in an interview after the competition, "*Jeopardy!* devotees know that buzzer skill is crucial—games between humans are more often won by the fastest thumb than the fastest brain. This advantage is only magnified when one of the 'thumbs' is an electromagnetic solenoid triggered by a microsecond-precise jolt of current."[7]

The human brain is truly the most sophisticated, elegant, biological piece of machinery ever known. And the good news is, you don't have to be a neuroscientist to understand some basic brain science. Have you ever been startled and experienced an adrenaline rush? Let's map out the brain circuit responsible for that heart-pounding event.

THE ALARM SYSTEM

What happens in the brain when we are afraid? Remember the little red metal square on the school-room wall with a piece of glass that reads, "Break in case of fire"? Just as the school has a fire alarm, so, too, our brain has an alarm switch called the amygdala (see the diagram on p. 7). When the fire alarm is activated at the school, its job is twofold: first to grab the attention of everyone in the building, and second to alert the 911 operator. Like that fire alarm, the amygdala both releases attention-getting adrenaline from the adrenal glands to the brain, and it alerts a sort of 911 operator to send out an urgent call. The brain's 911 operator is the hypothalamus, which is connected to the "radio tower" of the pituitary gland. Instead of radio waves, the pituitary gland transmits hormonal signals calling for the body's emergency response, which comes from the adrenal glands; they're the stress steroids known as glucocorticoids.

When emergency responders arrive at the school fire, there is a fire chief who assesses the extent of the blaze and how many responders are on the scene. When there are enough firefighters, the chief calls back to the 911 operator and reports that, even though the alarm is still going, the operator doesn't need to send any more.

Back in the brain, hippocampal neurons are the fire chief. They have glucocorticoid receptors that recognize the rise in stress hormones and signal back to the 911 operator (hypothalamus) saying, "Okay, you don't need to call any more responders (stress hormones)." Then, after the alarm has sounded, the brain's administrator, which is the dorsolateral prefrontal cortex (DLPFC, the part of the brain right behind the forehead), acting much like the school principal, evaluates whether there is real danger or whether it was a false alarm. If the administrator determines there is real danger, the alarm gets louder. If the administrator determines that there's been a "false alarm," everything calms down.

Here's an example of how this might work in your life. Imagine walking in a meadow with your family. As you step forward in the grass, out of the corner of your eye, you see something black and slithery by your feet. What happens? Your alarm (amygdala) fires and directly releases adrenaline from your adrenal glands to bring you to attention. The alarm also calls your 911 operator (hypothalamus), which immediately radios (sends hormone signals via the pituitary gland) for emergency responders (glucocoriticoids). The adrenal glands dispatch the responders and, in combination with the adrenaline, your heart rate rises, blood pressure shoots up, respirations increase, glucose is dumped into the bloodstream, blood is shunted away from your internal organs to your muscles, and you are primed to run out of there as fast as you can. This is the classic fight-or-flight response.

Then, after all of that happens, your "administrator" (DLPFC), the part of the brain right behind your forehead where you do your thinking and reasoning, turns on and says, "Hey, it's not a snake, it's just a rubber hose." And what happens? Everything immediately begins to calm down.

Or, imagine you hear a loud bang. Your alarm (amygdala) fires, causing the same cascade of excitatory events. The adrenaline surges through your system, bringing you to quick attention. Then your DLPFC evaluates the source of the noise. If this "administrator" concludes it was a car backfiring, you calm down. However, if it concludes a gunman is coming down the hall toward you, your alarm blares even louder and even greater surges of stress hormones flow through your body. One of the jobs of the prefrontal cortex is to process stimuli from your brain's emotional center and to either calm the system or put you squarely in fight-or-flight mode.[8]

Unfortunately, many people have difficulty calming their alarm circuitry, struggling with recurring or chronic fear. But why would that be? If God designed humanity in harmony with his law of love, what happened that so many are afraid and anxious?

THE ORIGIN OF FEAR

Imagine you are in a genuinely healthy, giving, other-centered, loving marriage. Your spouse is faithful, loyal, gracious and tenderly pours love on you. As you receive these signs of love, a corresponding chord is struck in your heart. Love flows through you back to your spouse as you give freely of yourself for his or her good. In this state, you experience the joy of God's design for human beings.

Now imagine that someone close to you—your mother, father, brother or sister, someone you also love and trust—comes to you and tells you a lie: your spouse is having an affair. You're even shown digitally altered photos showing your spouse in the arms of someone else. Even though there is absolutely no truth in it, even though your spouse is still loyal, faithful and true, if you *believe* the lie, something within you changes. The circle of love and trust is broken, and fear floods in!

Satan is the father of lies (Jn 8:44). He lied about God in heaven and he lied about God to Adam and Eve. They believed those lies, and the circle of love and trust was broken in the hearts and minds of our first parents. A cascade of destructive events followed. Notice the falling dominoes of destruction:

• Lies believed break the circle of love and trust.

Our first parents thought, "God, I don't believe you're good. I believe you are trying to keep me down, that you are hoarding power and control. Therefore, I don't trust you anymore."

• Broken love and trust results in fear and selfishness.

"God, now that I believe you are against me, I'm scared. I'm afraid of you and I can't trust you to watch out for me, so I have to take care of myself." Fear and selfishness are commonly known in the world today as "survival of the fittest," or the drive to survive, or "kill or be killed," or "watch out for me first." It is the polar opposite of giving, love or beneficence, and it is the infection that is destroying God's creation.

• Fear and selfishness result in acts of sin.

"I'd better get that fruit in order to exalt myself while I still can, before God gets rid of the tree and I lose my chance to get ahead."

• Acts of sin result in damage to mind, character and body—a terminal condition.

"The wages of sin is death" (Rom 6:23).

Once Adam and Eve believed the lies of the serpent, the circle of love and trust was broken in their hearts and minds. Believing Satan's mischaracterization of God, they no longer trusted him. From a neuroscience perspective, their prefrontal cortexes, rather than flowing with perfect love, activated the fear center (amygdala), inciting anxiety, insecurity and the desire to protect the self. In fear, Adam and Eve ran and hid. Their overactive, deregulated fear center further impaired their judgment, and they failed to think clearly and make healthy choices. They took matters into their own hands and not only ate the fruit, attempting to exalt themselves, but then also tried to repair their situation by making fig-leaf garments to cover up what they had done.

Eve believed the serpent and was afraid of God. Adam was afraid of losing Eve. In both cases, love was broken by a lie, and the brain, which God designed to grow and rewire itself based on the thoughts we think (we will explore this later) degenerated. The prefrontal cortex lost its governance and the fear center became inflamed. Love was suppressed and fear became the primary driving force in fallen humanity.

Those who live according to the sinful nature have their minds set on what that nature desires; but those who live in accordance with the Spirit have their minds set on what the Spirit desires. The mind of sinful man is death, but the mind controlled by the Spirit is life and peace; the sinful mind is hostile to God. It does not submit to God's law, nor can it do so. Those controlled by the sinful nature cannot please God. (Rom 8:5-8 NIV 1984)

Paul was saying that ever since Adam, humans have been born with their brains controlled by fear and selfishness; and such a state of disharmony with God's design for life results only in death. But when one trusts God, a change takes place: the prefrontal cortex is imbued with love and truth from the Holy Spirit, restoring God's balance, leading back to other-centered, peaceful living. On the other hand, the selfish, fear controlled brain is hostile to God and instead of submitting to love will be unable to please him. And this entire destructive cascade occurs because of believing lies about God.

Adam immediately demonstrated how utterly infected he was with the "watch out for me first" principle when he blamed Eve in an attempt to save himself, rather than offering himself to protect her. And because God gave Adam and Eve the ability to create beings in their image, every human descended from them is born infected with this terminal condition: our brains do not naturally function the way God designed.

Jesus taught that the acts of sin are the symptoms of a sin-sick heart when he said, "You have heard that it was said, 'Do not commit adultery.' But now I tell you: anyone who looks at a woman and wants to possess her is guilty of committing adultery with her in his heart." "For the mouth speaks what the heart is full of. A good person brings good things out of a treasure of good things; a bad person brings bad things out of a treasure of bad things." "For from your heart come the evil ideas which lead you to kill, commit adultery, and do other immoral things; to rob, lie, and slander others" (Mt 5:27-28; 12:34-35; 15:19 GNT).

What is Jesus saying? He's revealing to all of us that the acts of sin we so freely commit are symptoms or results of our sin-infected hearts and minds. The acts of sin are the inevitable consequences to the law of love being replaced with fear and selfishness in the heart. Our biological drive to put self first is so strong that without God's intervention, human beings are incapable of anything but fear-based, survival-driven selfishness. In fact, the freedom to love, the ability to choose to sacrifice self, all altruism is a manifestation of God's grace working in our hearts, in spite of ourselves—regardless of whether a person consciously acknowledges God or not. Because of Christ's victory (which we will explore later) and the work of the Holy Spirit, our hearts *can* choose to overcome our hereditary tendencies toward selfishness—but this will have to be a choice.

Now, what is the heart? Neurologically speaking the "heart" is the anterior cingulate cortex (ACC), the part of the brain right between your eyes and slightly back from your forehead. It is in this brain region where we experience empathy, compassion and love, and where we choose the right from the wrong.[9]

The part of the brain called the dorsolateral prefrontal cortex (DLPFC) is where we reason, strategize and plan. If you take your finger and touch the edge of your eyebrow closest to your ear and then move your finger straight up until you touch the natural hairline, the DLPFC lies beneath this point. Beneath the DLPFC, right above the top of the eye socket, is the orbital frontal cortex (OFC), and adjacent to the OFC toward the midline behind your nose is the ventral medial prefrontal cortex (VMPFC). Current brain science implicates the OFC and VMPFC as the most likely sites of the conscience. It is in the OFC and VMPFC where we experience the conviction of guilt and recognize socially inappropriate behavior, and from these regions the brain sends instructions to correct improper behavior.[10]

The DLPFC (reason) in combination with OFC and VMPFC (conscience) form the ability known as judgment. Interestingly, brain research has shown that when the VMPFC or conscience is active, the DLPFC or reason is less active, and vice versa. What this implies is that when our consciences are clear, we can reason and think more efficiently. But when we are involved in activities that violate God's law of love, the conscience impairs strategizing and planning. In other words, we cannot think clearly when we are guilt-ridden. In order for our judgment to work best, our consciences must be clear. This can only happen when we live in harmony with the law of love, which requires removing distorted God-concepts and coming back to a true knowledge of him. When we do so, the ACC (heart) grows stronger and calms or resolves the experience of guilt. Love is truly the basis of life.[11]

This amazing balance between reason (DLPFC) and conscience (VMPFC and OFC) was designed by God to enable finite beings to make healthy choices. When we contemplate activities that violate the law of love, the conscience (VMPFC) fires to alert us of danger and simultaneously impairs the ongoing planning of the destructive (sinful) action, while the OFC sends signals attempting to correct inappropriate behavior.

BRAIN BATTLE

Imagine that a person activates their DLPFC to plan how they can increase their income. If the idea, "I could grow some marijuana and sell it to the neighborhood kids" occurs, the VMPFC and OFC should begin to fire, bringing conviction that such a course is wrong, simultaneously impairing the functioning of the DLPFC and directing the person toward a different course. The healthy response would be to conclude, "No, that isn't a good idea," which would calm the VMPFC and OFC, and the DLPFC function would improve, especially as alternative actions are considered. When the idea of growing and selling tomatoes arises, the VMPFC and OFC remain quiet. No guilt is experienced, so the DLPFC stays unimpaired and healthy planning can be carried out.

Those who persist in the unhealthy (sinful/selfish) course, despite the firing of the conscience (VMPFC and OFC), may find greater difficulty extricating themselves from the destructive behaviors. This is due to the damaging effect that selfish and fear-based actions have on the ACC. It is in the ACC that the battle between love and self-ishness is ultimately won or lost. The fear-center impulses and the prefrontal cortex judgments meet at the ACC. Here we must come to a decision and resolve the internal tension.[12]

God's methods of love and truth strengthen the ACC and calm the fear circuits. This means that the more clearly we embrace love-based God-concepts and act altruistically, the healthier our brains become; and on the other hand, the more fear-inducing our God-concept is, the more selfish our actions and the more damage occurs. Because the fear circuits of the brain produce powerful emotions and can lead to impulsive decision making, our emotions are not designed to be in charge of our actions.[13]

Yes, God designed us to experience pleasure and deeply powerful emotions, but this is meant to be in harmony with healthy prefrontal cortex action. Have you ever had the experience of struggling with a problem, puzzle or difficult question, and after days of study and contemplation the "light" finally went on and you formulated the answer? How did you feel? Was there a "pleasurable" sensation? That positive emotion was because the prefrontal cortex activated the brain's emotional system as God designed.

When you experience pleasure in a loving relationship, exhila-ration at a beautiful sunset, and that emotional "high" after a five-mile run, you are experiencing healthy activation of your emotional brain regions as God designed them to function. The problem occurs when the emotions control the ACC to override good judgment and we use our energies to satisfy what our selfish desires want. This is the problem with fear-based decision making; the emotion circuits dominate, and selfishness is chosen instead of love.

Our acts of self-indulgence then further damage our brain, body, character and relationships, ultimately resulting in our death. This is our inherited condition from Adam; this is our diagnosis. We are born infected with fear and selfishness corrupting our entire being, with brains out of balance, with overdeveloped fear circuits and underdeveloped love circuits, with minds that no longer know God nor operate on his law of love. Without divine intervention, this condition is terminal, for life is only compatible with the law of love.

A LIE BELIEVED

In March 2008, after two years of investigation, prosecution and deliberation, fifty-three-year-old John White was sentenced to prison for aggravated manslaughter. John White admitted to shooting Daniel Cicciaro, a seventeen-year-old neighbor and friend of John's son, Aaron.

How could such a tragedy happen? How could the circle of friendship get broken? What could cause neighbor to shoot neighbor? A lie was told. A lie was believed. The circle of love and trust was broken.

Here's what happened. Michael Longo, a friend of John White's son, Aaron, logged onto Aaron White's MySpace account and sent a message threatening to rape a teenage girl who was a close friend of Daniel Cicciaro. Michael Longo said, under testimony, that he did this as a practical joke. But Daniel Cicciaro believed the threat was real, so he gathered three friends to deal with the situation.

He called Aaron White repeatedly. He threatened Aaron, calling him racially derogatory slurs. He told Aaron the four young men were on the way to his house to kill him. Aaron woke his father, and as the four men approached the house, Aaron and John—both armed with guns—went out onto the porch, where they argued with the four young men. The meeting culminated in John White shooting Daniel Cicciaro in the face.

Daniel Cicciaro believed he was protecting his friend from being raped. John White believed he was protecting his son from being killed. Both believed they were doing what was right, protecting another. Why did this tragedy happen? A lie was believed! Once the circle of love and trust was broken, fear and selfishness inflamed in the heart.

OUR TERMINAL CONDITION IS NOT OUR FAULT

Imagine that an HIV-infected man and an HIV-infected woman have a child, and that child is born HIV-infected. What did the child do wrong? Nothing! Just like you and me, we didn't do anything wrong to be born in this terminally selfish state. It isn't our fault we are born with brains out of balance. But just like that baby, even though it did nothing wrong, it still suffers from a condition that, unless cured, will kill it. That is our situation as well. We are not born guilty; we are born terminal: "dead in your transgressions and sins" (Eph 2:1). We are born with brains that naturally fire the alarm center, impair the prefrontal cortex and seek to protect self at the expense of others.

Humanity was created by God to operate on perfect other-centered, outward-moving love, giving in beneficial action toward others. As long as Adam and Eve were in perfect harmony with the law of love, they would not die. But to sin is to break the law (1 Jn 3:4). Sin is severing the law of love. Just as cutting its throat kills the animal, or throwing the switch turns off the lights, or removing money from circulation destroys the economy, when the law of love is broken, the only possible outcome without divine intervention is ruin and death. "The wages of sin is death" (Rom 6:23). "Sin, when it is full-grown, gives birth to death" (Jas 1:15).

But why? Because a brain in which the fear circuits rule is cut off from God, our very source of life. Only love, coming from God, is capable of freeing us from fear.

Brain-imaging studies have demonstrated that the more time a person spends in communion with the God of love, the more developed the ACC becomes. Not only that, the person experiences decreases in stress hormones, blood pressure, heart rate and risk of untimely death. Even in our mortal and defective bodies, love is healing. Conversely, the more time spent contemplating an angry, wrathful, fear-inducing deity, the more damage to the brain and the more rapidly one's health declines, leading to early death.[14]

THE GIVER OF LIFE

Jesus came so that we might have life and have it more abundantly, here and now, as we anticipate the day that the mortal life puts on immortality (Jn 10:10; 1 Cor 15:53). The abundant life is the life of love, which only occurs when we replace the twisted versions of God with truth, enabling God's love to flow through us to others. And it is in the prefrontal cortex that we comprehend truth, experience God's love and altruistically love others.

As I continued in my imagination that day, I saw that tragic event when the lies about God were believed and the floodgate of ruin and death opened. The circle of giving, the principle of other-centered goodness, was no longer the rule of life on planet Earth. When Adam believed the lies about God and broke the circle of love and trust, his rule of love changed to one of fear and selfishness—and nature followed. The drive to survive—kill or be killed, Satan's antagonistic principle of me-first—infected the entire world. The heavenly hosts mourned as they saw the corruption spread. The earth began to change. Flowers faded and died, leaves fell from trees, and decay emerged. Animals began attacking each other. The strong preyed on the weak. Thorns, thistles and noxious plants appeared. Brother turned against brother as anger, jealousy and hatred obliterated love from the heart. God began to grieve, nature groaned—the infection was spreading (Rom 8:19-22).

3

The Infection of Fear

Those who love to be feared fear to be loved,
and they themselves are more afraid than anyone,
for whereas other men fear only them,
they fear everyone.

SAINT FRANCIS DE SALES

VINCE WAS WHAT YOU MIGHT call pitiful. He came to see me depressed, unhappy and contemplating suicide. Vince attracted women like honey attracts bees. Then in his forties, he was athletic, trim and strong as a mountain mustang. He was considered handsome by most, and the business he owned was financially secure. Despite all his apparent success, though, Vince was never happy, never at peace and never able to maintain a healthy relationship.

He'd struggled through a long history of failed relationships, each following a predictable pattern. Vince would pursue a woman and, usually, win her affection. But once the two were in a relationship, his fear and insecurity would take over. He doubted whether he deserved the woman he was with. He was afraid no one could really love him, and his anxiety inevitably contaminated every romance in a variety of ways.

Vince would shower his girlfriends with gifts, notes, phone calls, and emails—not because he wanted to give but as a means to get them to praise and admire him. Initially his girlfriends were flattered and swept off their feet. Over time, they invariably became exhausted and tired of his constant need for praise, attention and admiration.

But of course it wasn't just tokens of affection: Vince's fear had an ugly side too. He was violently jealous and saw threats at every turn. If his girlfriend chose to study for an exam rather than go out with him, he would accuse her of wanting to go out with other guys. If her phone rang and she didn't answer, he suspected she was getting calls from other men. If they were out and another man looked her way, he would confront the onlooker, embarrassing his girlfriend. So insecure, so fearful, so constantly afraid was he that he monitored his girlfriends' phones, behavior, emails and friends. Inescapably, every relationship ended the same with Vince being unceremoniously dumped.

THE FEAR FACTOR

Fear is an intruder, an unnatural invader, like a flesh-eating bacteria—ravaging and deforming all creation. As soon as Adam believed the lies about God and the circle of love and trust was broken, fear infected the human heart. Fueled by fear and selfishness, the imagination of men ran wild and created every distorted, twisted and perverted idea about God, which only incited more fear (Jer 17:9; Rom 1:18-21; 2 Cor 10:5).

Today fear is constantly with us, stalking us, hiding in the shadows of our minds. We may beat it back for brief moments, but it lurks in the darkness of our hearts. It doesn't wait for an invitation; it barges into our lives, trampling our world like cattle tromping daisies. I'm not talking about adaptive alertness, which comes when the house is burning, a bear is approaching or you near the edge of a cliff. No, fear born of sin is a noxious uneasiness boiling in our unconscious minds, threatening to destroy our every happiness. We run from it, but it propels us ever forward as we search, grope and hope for relief. But fear only leads us into more pain.

Fear is part of the infection of sin. It leads us away from God, away from healing, away from peace into further self-destruction. Several years ago I read about a high-school chemistry instructor and two of her senior students who were arrested and found guilty of arson and insurance fraud. The chemistry professor was several months behind on her car payments and the vehicle was about to be repossessed. The two senior students were failing her class.

She proposed a deal: If the two failing students stole her car and burned it, she would file an insurance claim to avoid having the car repossessed and her credit ruined. In exchange, she would give them passing grades in chemistry. They carried out her plan but were caught. All three were sent to prison. Fear impairs our judgment, paralyzes our reason and leads us down the path of selfishness.

THE MANY FACES OF FEAR

Fear comes in many sizes and shapes. At one end of the fear spectrum is the megalomaniac—the type of fear demonstrated by Hitler, Stalin, Castro and other despots. Their rise to power was fueled by fear: fear of the Jews, Gypsies, Slavs, Christians, capitalism and freedom itself. Such thugs of history were consumed with fear, but rather than eradicate it, they embraced it, joined their hearts to it and became one with it. Fear became their weapon against society, splitting, dividing, conquering and destroying. These ambassadors of evil, with hearts and minds so shaped by anti-love, created mangled societies battered by fear. And history is clear: where fear abounds, death quickly follows.

On the other end of the spectrum from the megalomaniac is the human "mouse." Afraid of rejection, fearful of embarrassment, terrified of criticism, people made meek by fear abase themselves into doormats walked on by the entire world. They never say no, never stand up, and never set boundaries because they are controlled by fear of what others might say and how others might respond or think.

In between these two extremes exist all manner of fear-ridden apparitions morphing insecurity into their own unique survival mechanism—the playground bully, the proud, the arrogant, the racist, the bigoted and the sexist. Here you'll also find the alcoholic, drug addict, sex addict and shopaholic; the religionist, cultist and separatist; the philanderer, the liar, the cheater and fraud—each motivated by fear, each seeking some way to protect self, promote self or advance self. But rather than surviving, rather than healing, rather than growing, all are slowly dying and destroying others in the process. Life, health and happiness are only found where love flows free. And love only flows free where the truth about God is known![1]

OUT OF BALANCE

The constant firing of the anxiety system occurs in brains out of balance and is an overreaction to environmental stimuli. Because of sin, all of our brains are out of balance and we all experience, far too frequently, the effects of out-of-control stress, the amygdala firing. Evolutionary biologists would suggest that the fight-or-flight response is a very adaptive reaction to promote survival in the face of immediate crisis. But it is the firing of this alarm system that damages the brain, impairs healthy thinking and abuses the body. The longer the alarm fires, the more pronounced the damage.

If the alarm (amygdala) doesn't turn off, even though our fire chief (hippocampus) is holding our 911 operator (hypothalamus) in check, the constant stress impairs physical growth by shunting blood and energy away from our internal organs to the muscles. Further, our immune system is impaired and our prefrontal cortex becomes paralyzed. This is why people under high stress are more vulnerable to infections, colds and other illnesses, and why people perform so poorly on examinations when they are anxious and fearful.[2]

FEAR AND LOVE ARE INVERSELY PROPORTIONAL

Here's the bottom line: When fear increases, love, growth, development and healthy thinking decrease. When love increases, not only does fear decrease, but growth, development and healthy thinking all improve. Fear and love are inversely proportional. It is in our prefrontal cortex that we experience healthy love, compassion, altruism, empathy, reasoning capacity, judgment, the ability to worship, conscientiousness, morality, and the ability to plan, organize and problem solve. Whereas, fear, insecurity, selfishness, anger, rage, lust, jealousy, envy and aggression arise from our constantly stimulated limbic systems.[3]

Which brings us back to Vince. Vince was chronically insecure, and the more fear he experienced, the more his amygdala fired, impairing his prefrontal-cortex function. Having never known healthy love, his prefrontal cortex was dominated by the impulses of his limbic system. Vince did not act in gracious, loving, compassionate and mature ways toward his girlfriends. Therefore, his relationships always failed, and the failed relationships caused Vince to think in negative ways about himself and others. His negative thought processes created unhealthy neural circuits in his prefrontal cortex, which only fired the amygdala more intensely, further impairing healthy prefrontal-cortex function. He was caught in a painful, vicious downward cycle. This process damages the brain and, if it is not stopped, eventually the ability to think in healthy ways is completely lost. But, how does all of this get started?

THE DEVELOPING BRAIN

One possible avenue for anxiety to be instigated is a prebirth effect on the brain. Brain development begins in utero. Unfortunately, since any unusually high stress causes the body to release stress hormones (glucocorticoids), if this occurs during a woman's pregnancy those stress hormones cross the placental barrier and alter the developing fetal brain. They impair the "braking system" on the amygdala of the growing brain, which means that a child born to a high-stress mother will have a brain less capable of calming itself and turning off the alarm circuitry. Such children will start life from a baseline that is more anxious and fearful than they would otherwise have experienced.[4]

After birth, a baby's brain contains hundreds of millions more neurons at birth than it will have when it is eight years of age. For the first eight years of life the brain is busy killing off neurons by the hundreds of millions. At first this doesn't sound too productive. But think of it like Michelangelo's block of marble before he begins work on it, and then think of the same block of marble after he has transformed it into a wondrous work of art. When the artist finishes, he has less marble, but he has a masterpiece. The brain comes into the world prepared to be acted on by education, environment and experience. Neurons by the millions are waiting to be retained, strengthened and expanded. But those neural circuits that are not used become pruned, deleted or reassigned.[5]

Maybe you have heard case reports of children who were neglected, abused or abandoned and did not have normal language exposure. Such neglected children never learn to speak normally. One case is that of "Genie" who, at approximately twenty months of age, was locked inside a room and spent the next eleven years of her life in isolation. When she was rescued at age thirteen she was profoundly disabled and, despite intensive rehabilitative efforts, never learned to speak effectively. Another case was Kamala, reportedly found living with wolves by missionary J. A. Singh when the child was eight years of age. She could not speak but made inarticulate howling noises, walked on all fours, and lapped food like a dog. Despite living for nine more years, she never learned to speak more than fifty words.[6]

These tragic cases demonstrate normal human brain processes—neural circuits that are not used either fail to develop or are pruned and deleted, but those circuits that are used are strengthened and expanded. This happens throughout the entire brain. Therefore, activities that repeatedly and regularly excite or fire the amygdala (alarm) during childhood will enhance its development and impair growth of the prefrontal cortex.

ENTERTAINMENT AND THE DEVELOPING BRAIN

One of the unheralded factors contributing to the rise of fear and psychiatric disorders is the high prevalence of theatrical entertainment, including television watching, especially among children. Theatrical entertainment refers to programming designed, through pretense or artificial enactments, to cause emotional reactions, while for the most part disengaging critical reasoning. Earlier we explored normal brain development. We discovered that during the first eight years of life, the brain is busy killing off synaptic connections by the hundreds of millions. Neural circuits that are used are kept. Those left idle either fail to develop or are deleted. Understanding this normal physiological process is the key to understanding the devastation theatrical TV has wrought on the brain.

Theatrical programming, which is not to be confused with educational programming, has as its primary effect to fire the limbic system while simultaneously diminishing prefrontal cortex activity. Theatrical entertainment is designed to get an emotional response from the audience, and the more powerful the emotional reaction the "better" the program. Such programs want to get you to laugh, or cry, or be afraid, aroused, angry, irritated or frustrated, while simultaneously turning off your critical thinking.[7]

I have some friends who loved to watch the popular television program called 24, but not when I was around because I would usually say something like, "This is stupid." One season's storyline went something like this: An illegal alien terrorist entered America. He (and/or his cronies) gained access to a top-secret, high-security military base and stole a nuclear weapon along with its arming codes. He then sneaked into a different facility and stole a stealth cruise missile. Then, at a remote farm in the Midwest, he and his technicians paired the two elements together, programmed the missile, fired it and destroyed a U.S. city—all in a twenty-four-hour period. Think about that for a moment.

When I dismissed the plot as ridiculous, my friends responded, "You're not supposed to think about it. You're not supposed to reason. You're supposed to suspend logic." In other words, to enjoy the program, I had to turn off my reasoning (DLPFC) and then allow my limbic system to run ungoverned and experience the roller coaster of anxious emotions the show was designed to elicit.

Theatrical programming has a similar impact on most human brains, but children between birth and eight years are particularly vulnerable because of the massive modification of neural circuitry occurring during this time. Studies have shown that the more theatrical entertainment children view during the first eight years of life, the greater their risk of attention, focus and concentration problems (dysfunction of the prefrontal cortex), and the higher the rates of violence, impulsive behavior, sexual acting out, and increased anxiety and mood problems.

Sadly, many parents, the mainstream media and even church groups have wrongly concluded that this problem is entirely content-driven. The old adage "garbage in, garbage out" has been used by many a well-meaning preacher to discourage bad content. While it is absolutely appropriate to avoid bad content, the problem with theatrical entertainment is not primarily content-driven. The issue is a neural-developmental one. In other words, watching G-rated theatrical entertainment will still damage the developing brain.

VIOLENT LINK

Dr. Brandon Centerwall did the seminal study on this issue, published in the *Journal of the American Medical Association*, in 1992. He wanted to determine if there was a link between television watching and increased violence in society. This would indicate that a dysfunction in brain circuitry as aggression, rage and anger arises from the limbic system while the prefrontal cortex exercises self-control and restraint. Thus increasing violence indicates the loss of prefrontal-cortex control of limbic-system impulses. Dr. Centerwall used a clear indicator of violence—homicide rates before and after the introduction of TV into society. He chose three countries in which to conduct his research: the United States, Canada and South Africa.

The United States and Canada allowed the introduction of TV into their countries in 1945, but South Africa did not allow TV until 1974. Canada was included because Canada has strict gun-control laws, and if a rise in homicide rates was seen in the United States, Dr. Centerwall didn't want easy access to guns to detract from the impact of television watching. And to guard against apartheid racist policies of South Africa skewing the findings, only white-on-white homicide was measured.

The results were astounding. Between 1945 and 1974, after the introduction of television, homicide rates in Canada increased 92 percent. In the United States, murder rates increased 93 percent, but in South Africa during the same time period, white on white homicide *decreased* 7 percent. But here's the kicker: Dr. Centerwall examined white-on-white homicide in South Africa from 1974 to 1987, after the introduction of television, and shockingly, homicide rates soared by 130 percent.[8]

What type of programming was on television in the United States between 1945 and 1974? *Howdy Doody, Leave It to Beaver, I Love Lucy, Car 54, Gilligan's Island, Lassie, Rin Tin Tin, The Lone Ranger*—shows like that. What rating would all of these shows receive? A G rating. Yet homicide rates still increased 92 percent in Canada and 93 percent in the United States. When the content worsened after 1974, the homicide rates jumped by 130 percent. If television watching is playing a role in societal violence, it seems that content is a magnifier of the problem but not the core issue.

In 2007 Frederick Zimmerman and Dimitri Christakis confirmed that educational television watching in children over the age of two did not worsen attention problems, but both nonviolent and violent theatrical programming did.[9]

The primary issue is neural developmental. Overstimulation of the limbic system by theatrical entertainment—while decreasing the usage of the prefrontal cortex during the developmental years—results in children growing up with brains out of balance. When adolescence is reached and the hormones surge, the limbic system becomes inflamed and emotions become unstable. Without prefrontal cortexes properly developed to process and restrain the limbic system, and with overly developed emotional centers, such teens not only have higher risks of attention problems but are more likely to be moody, impulsive and aggressive, and to suffer increased anxiety and emotional volatility leading to sexual promiscuity and violence. There's also a corresponding increased risk of alcohol and illegal drug use in attempts to chemically calm themselves.

Music videos, which activate limbic circuits, have also been associated with increased violence and destructive behavior. Research by Gina Wingwood and others documented that adolescents who were exposed to rap music videos were 3 times more likely to have hit a teacher; more than 2.5 times as likely to have been arrested; 2 times as likely to have had multiple sexual partners; and more than 1.5 times as likely to have acquired a new sexually transmitted disease, used drugs and used alcohol over the twelve-month follow-up period. Other research has documented that watching pop music videos increased the risk of adolescent alcohol consumption by 31 percent.[10]

CHILDHOOD STRESS CHANGES THE BRAIN

While theatrical entertainment negatively impacts brain development, childhood traumas are even more damaging. Dr. Andrea Danese and her team followed over 800 individuals for thirty-two years to determine the impact childhood stress has on mental and physical health. They identified three measures of childhood stress:

overt physical or sexual abuse, neglect, and socioeconomic deprivation. The research team categorized people into three groups,
those with none of the three adverse events during childhood, those
with one adverse event and those with two or more. Then, over the
next thirty-two years, the researchers documented who developed
depression, metabolic problems such as diabetes, increased inflammation, and overall increased risk for disease. The results demonstrated that the more childhood stress the higher incidence of
depression, inflammation (the implication of which we'll see below)
and metabolic illnesses later in life. The study concluded: "Children
exposed to adverse psychosocial experiences have enduring emotional, immune, and metabolic abnormalities that contribute to
explaining their elevated risk for age-related disease."[11]

Children who are raised in high-stress, low-nurturing or abusive
environments experience overdevelopment of the fear/emotion
centers and underdevelopment of the reason, love and judgment
centers. They experience greater levels of stress hormones throughout
development, which results in greater vulnerability to a variety of
chronic disease states, including depression, inflammatory diseases
and metabolic problems. Because of these brain changes, such individuals have difficulty with empathy, compassion, trust, altruistic love,
sympathizing with others, patience and overall healthy relationships.[12]

This was one of Vince's problems. He not only had bad examples
given to him in childhood, but the high stress he experienced caused
brain changes that made healthy love and healthy thinking more
difficult to experience. Vince's overly sensitive amygdala and unhealthy prefrontal cortex caused him to anticipate injury, slight and
rejection when no real threat existed. Therefore, he was overly controlling in an attempt to avoid getting hurt, rejected or abandoned.

Vince's battle between love and fear is not his alone. Every human
being descended from Adam and Eve is born infected with fear and
selfishness—fear of failure, fear of what others think, fear of not
getting that job, fear of not getting that guy or girl, fear of not getting

that grade, fear of not being loved, fear of being alone, fear, fear, fear!

According to the National Institute of Mental Health, anxiety disorders are the most common mental health problem in America, affecting 28.8 percent of adults at some point in their lives—and the rate of anxiety disorder incidence appears to be on the rise. When the fear center of the brain (amygdala) is activated and is not calmed, it triggers a cascade of caustic events, which ravages our bodies and brains. The sympathetic nervous system activates the release of stress hormones (glucocorticoids and adrenaline) and inflammatory factors (cytokines). The inflammatory factors wreak havoc in the body increasing illness, metabolic problems and pain.[13]

FERTILIZER FOR THE BRAIN

The continual elevation of these inflammatory factors eventually react back on the brain, causing the suppression of genes that produce proteins called neurotrophic factors. One such protein is brain-derived neurotrophic factor (BDNF). "Brain derived," meaning that the brain makes it; "neurotrophic," referring to something that makes neurons grow strong. Think of BDNF as fertilizer for your neurons. When this protein is available, the neurons that get it grow stronger and send out more connections to other neurons, increasing brain circuits. The brain even makes new neurons under the influence of such proteins. With this protein available in the right brain regions, we can learn faster and easier. When this protein and other proteins like it are unavailable, the brain stops making new neurons and the neurons we have begin to wither and die.

In the brain, the white supporting cells surround the neurons like an astronaut's space suit. Just as the space suit provides a safe environment for the astronaut, the white cells surround the neurons, dendrites, axons and the connections called synapses, bathing the neurons in rich nutritional fluids that the neurons like. Not only do the neurons themselves make BDNF, but the supporting cells also make BDNF, helping to keep the neurons healthy.

But the persistent rise in inflammatory factors, resulting from chronic fear and anxiety, cause several problems for the brain. First, they damage the white brain cells that provide the protection and support for the neurons. Second, stress—the fight-or-flight response—shuts down growth by suppressing growth factors like BDNF. This impairs new learning and development.

The chronic stress signal causes a message to be transmitted to the DNA in the brain cells—both the neurons and the white cells—turning off the gene that produces BDNF. Once this gene is turned off, brain volume begins to shrink in the hippocampus and parts of the prefrontal cortex. Such brain changes correlate with disorders like major depression.[14]

The good news is that many brain regions remain changeable throughout life, thanks to a condition called neuroplasticity. This is particularly true of the prefrontal cortex. As we exercise healthy neural circuits, these circuits develop, strengthen and expand. Conversely, the brain prunes unhealthy circuits when we leave them idle.

GOD'S METHODS AND PERSONAL APPLICATION

When God's methods for increasing brain health and nurturing mental stability are applied, the brain circuits of the prefrontal cortex actually grow stronger and, despite previous damage, healing ensues. Healthy connections grow and develop. If you are someone who has suffered abuse during childhood, or if you've struggled with an overly active limbic system resulting in too much aggression, irritability, impatience, anger, lust, selfishness, fear or insecurity, don't be discouraged. God's methods bring healing.

And what are God's methods? Truth, love and freedom. In order to be beneficial, treatment must be applied; truth is only beneficial when it is understood, believed and applied. So examine the three threads of evidence: Scripture, testable laws in nature and experience. Do you see harmony among the three threads, demonstrating that humanity currently struggles with fear and selfishness? Does the evidence confirm that selfish exploitation is destructive? And does the evidence support God's methods are healing and restorative? God's methods would include but not be limited to:

• Worshiping a God of love and rejecting God-concepts that induce fear.

• Regular meditation on some aspect of God's character of love, at least fifteen minutes per day.

• Being truthful and eliminating falsehood of any kind from the mind. This is particularly important for those who have suffered abuse. Abused children, because of the level of brain development, will misconstrue the meaning of the abuse and internalize distortions about themselves. Typical falsehoods include such ideas as, "I'm ugly. I'm gross. I'm nasty, dirty, disgusting and unlovable." All such distortions must be replaced with the truth. Think about it. If you walked in on an adult man abusing a six-year-old child, would you ever think, "That's a disgusting six-year-old"? Never! But the child invariably walks away feeling awful about him- or herself. While the facts of history cannot be changed, the adult who has suffered abuse can reevaluate the historic event and apply the truth, that the awful feelings once experienced belong to the event, not to the self. The application of truth is healing.

• Live to give. Actively seek to help others; get involved with some ministry or volunteer activity.

• Establish relationships with people of loving and mature character, and terminate destructive and exploitive relationships.[15]

• Trust God with your life and your life's outcomes. Choose to fulfill your known responsibilities in harmony with a clear conscience and God's will, and then *trust* God with how things turn out. One of the greatest sources of worry and fear is trying to *make* life turn out the way we want, rather than simply choosing what is right in governance of self and trusting God with the outcome. (Consider the three worthies on the plain of Dura recorded in Daniel. Bow to the idol or not, that was their choice. How things turned out, they could not control. But too often in such circumstances we don't focus on our known responsibility but instead focus on what will happen as a result of our choice—and then modify our choice to affect the outcome. If we were on that plain, knowing it was wrong to bow but not wanting to go into a fiery furnace, when the music played might we have bent down to tie our shoe?)

• Live in harmony with the physical design protocols for life, such as regular sleep, drink plenty of water, exercise mind and body regularly, avoid toxins, and eat a balanced diet.

• When mistakes are made, resolve guilt as soon as possible, forgive those who mistreat you, and don't hold to anger or grudges as such emotions activate the body's inflammatory cascade.

• Resolve fear, as unremedied fear truly destroys.

It is love that heals and restores, but genuine love is only experienced when lies about God are removed.

4

Freedom to Love

*The greatest dangers to liberty lurk in
insidious encroachment by men of zeal,
well-meaning but without understanding.*

LOUIS D. BRANDEIS

LET ME TELL YOU ABOUT "Joe." Sadly, I don't "know" him, even though I have gone to church with him for more than twenty years. I don't know him because, even though he is a living, flesh-and-blood human being, in a very real sense he is only a shadow. And shadows don't have substance. Shadows don't have individuality or identity.

It was more than forty years ago when Joe married Martha. They were both Christians belonging to a conservative denomination and were active in their local church. Joe was an intelligent man, a skilled craftsman, a carpenter in high demand because of the quality of his work.

When they first married, Joe enjoyed social gatherings, where he would share his experiences, talk with others and participate in activities. Joe was involved in men's ministries and volunteered his talents, time and ability to assist those less fortunate. But early in the marriage things began to change.

At home his wife was unhappy. She became demanding and was jealous of his time spent helping others. She began to complain, whine and criticize. She would pout, throw tantrums, yell and withhold affection. Initially Joe tried to console her, to reason with her and calm her, but nothing changed. So Joe began to limit his activities. He stopped volunteering and stopped meeting with friends.

Over the years he withdrew more and more in order to please his wife, in order to keep her happy. In public he stopped socializing. He no longer initiated conversations. When someone asked him a question, he looked to his wife for permission to speak. Slowly, gradually, almost imperceptibly Joe faded away. He lost himself. His prefrontal cortex was damaged. His individuality was eroded so all that remained was a mere shadow.

THE LAW OF LIBERTY

God runs his universe on certain principles, certain fundamental laws, certain constants on which life is designed to operate. As we have seen, the primary law is love, which emanates from the heart of God and is the base code for life. But love cannot exist in an atmosphere without freedom. This is the subject of *Could It Be This Simple? A Biblical Model for Healing the Mind*, in which I lay out what I call the "law of liberty."

Whenever liberty is violated, three predictable consequences occur: (1) love is always damaged and will eventually be destroyed; (2) a desire to rebel is instilled in the heart and, if one has the option to restore freedom but instead chooses to remain violated, then (3) individuality is slowly eroded and the person becomes, like Joe, a mere shadow.

SUBMERGED UNDER ANOTHER

Joe's problem was similar to Lynda's. Lynda was a thirty-six-year-old patient referred to me by her counselor. She complained of panic epi-

sodes, depression and anxiety. She worried all the time and complained of inability to think clearly or make decisions. She maintained
a chronic fear of failure, fear of rejection and fear of making mistakes.

She had even been hospitalized on several occasions for suicidal thinking and disorganized behavior, and she had been
treated with fourteen different medications over the years, with no
significant improvement.

Lynda told me she had married a man who was domineering,
controlling and demanding. He monitored her every move. He gave
her money only to use as he directed. When money was given for
groceries, her husband required that she give him receipts showing
every penny spent and returning any change to him. She could not
use the phone without permission, and was forbidden from talking
to old friends or developing new ones. This man dictated her every
move. If she tried to have any initiative or individuality, he would
verbally assault her, criticize her and accuse her of being an un-
loving wife. And now she was having panic attacks.

Imagine someone pushing your head under water and holding you
there. Maybe if you thought it was a joke, it wouldn't be too bad for the
first five seconds. But how would you feel after fifteen seconds? Thirty?
Sixty? With every passing second the anxiety would build until abject
panic set in. You would either get your head above water or die! That
is a very good picture of what was happening to Lynda. Her identity,
her individuality, her unique personhood was submerged under that
of her husband's. She was being suffocated as a person. She was dying
on the inside. She would either regain her autonomy or lose herself
completely and become a mere shadow of her husband.

GOD'S STANDARD, OUR SPIRITUAL WEAPON

Violate liberty, and love is always damaged. Eventually it will even
be destroyed. A desire to rebel is instilled in the heart, but if one sur-
renders to violations long enough, individuality is shattered so that
only a shadow remains. Love cannot exist in an atmosphere without

freedom. This law is not enacted or legislated; it is one of the principles on which life is designed to operate, and our health and happiness are dependent on harmony with it.

If you have doubts about the reality of this law, then please test it.
It is essential you are convinced. Test it on your significant other. For
a day, try restricting his or her liberties. Tell your special other where
he can go, what she must wear, when he can use the phone, how
much money can be spent. See for yourself what happens to love.[1]

Conversely, if you are in a relationship in which freedoms have
been abused, begin to breathe in liberty and see if love revives. Begin
to promote the health, welfare and happiness of your spouse.
Promote his or her dreams, goals and aspirations, and watch love
blossom and grow.[2]

Once we understand that this law is real—that it works, that it is a
constant, that it never changes—then we have something measurable, tangible, reliable and predictable. We have another standard
against which we can test our theories, our doctrines and our beliefs
about God. We now have a second tool to separate the healthy from
the damaging views of God, for God will never violate his own character of love, which means God does not take away freedom or operate contrary to the law of liberty.

This standard, this law, is one of the spiritual weapons we can wield
in our warfare against evil forces. Notice the central issue in the war:

> For though we live in the world, we do not wage war as the
> world does. The weapons we fight with are not the weapons
> of the world. On the contrary, they have divine power to de-
> molish strongholds. We demolish arguments and every pre-
> tension that sets itself up against *the knowledge of God*, and
> we take captive every thought to make it obedient to Christ.
> (2 Cor 10:3-5, emphasis mine)

We are actually at war against anything that sets itself up against the
knowledge of God. The war is over the truth about God, who God is,

and what he is like. Can he be trusted? Satan lied about God, and lies believed break the circle of love and trust. Love cannot flow where lies are retained, so we war against those lies in order to restore trust and reopen the channels of love.

HOW OUR THOUGHTS REWIRE OUR BRAINS

Why is knowing the truth about God so critical, and what impact does it have on the brain? God created us in his image, with the ability to adapt and change based on our choices and experiences. When we believe lies about God those false beliefs actually damage us, change our neural circuits, and warp our minds and characters. Conversely, when we receive the truth we are also changed, conformed back into the image of God through the working of his Spirit. Brain science has given us some insights into the amazing pathways through which our thoughts actually change our brains.

In chapter 3 we explored proteins called neurotrophic factors, one being Brain Derived Neurotrophic Factor (BDNF), a protein acting like fertilizer for our brain cells. Along with similar proteins produced in our glia (white brain cells) and blood vessels, BDNF causes the neurons to grow stronger, branch out, connect and even form new neurons. But our DNA does not directly "code for" BDNF—in other words, BDNF doesn't leave the DNA as BDNF but as a precursor protein called proBDNF. But proBDNF is not inactive. In fact, its effects are opposite BDNF. While BDNF is fertilizer for neurons, proBDNF is like weed killer to neurons. If proBDNF binds to dendrites, axons or neurons, it will kill them. The critical issue to determine whether a neuron or neural circuit gets BDNF (fertilizer) or proBDNF (weed killer) is the presence of an enzyme that cleaves or cuts the longer chain molecule (proBDNF) into the shorter molecule BDNF. If the enzyme is present, BDNF is available and the circuit grows stronger. If the enzyme is not present, proBDNF is not cleaved and thus proBDNF prunes the circuit back.[3]

What determines if a neural circuit will have the enzyme to

cleave proBDNF into BDNF? It's the activity of the neural circuit itself. If the circuit is utilized, active and firing, it produces the enzyme that cleaves proBDNF into BDNF, and the circuit grows stronger, recruiting more neurons and making new connections. If, however, the circuit is idle, it doesn't produce the enzyme and proBDNF is not cleaved. Therefore, over time, the circuit is slowly pruned back.[4]

Consider taking a foreign-language course. Those first few days using brute-force memory to learn words cause new synaptic connections to form. Each day of practice causes more firing of the newly forming neural circuit. This activity within the neural circuit produces the enzyme necessary to cleave proBDNF into BDNF; and the neurons branch faster, new neurons are recruited, new connections made, and your ability to speak the language improves. Over the course of several years of speaking this new language the circuitry expands to the point that not only does vocabulary increase but syntax and pronunciation also improves.

But then you stop speaking that language, and twenty years goes by. What happens to your proficiency? The circuit isn't fired; the enzyme which cleaves proBDNF isn't produced, so slowly, over the years, the neural circuitry corresponding to this language is pruned.

What if you practiced speaking the foreign language in your imagination, but didn't actually speak it out loud—would the circuit degrade? Functional brain imaging would indicate that it would not, or at least not as quickly. Now let's apply this to emotional health. In 2007 brain research revealed that the same brain circuits that activate to painful stimuli also activate when people *imagine* painful stimuli. In 2000, Karl Herholz and Wolf-Dieter Heiss discovered that stroke patients who merely imagined moving an affected limb *actually* activated the corresponding motor circuits in their brains. This is the concept of visualization in artistic and athletic performance: brain studies have shown that when musicians imagine playing a piece of music, the same motor pathways activate as if they were actually playing their instrument, even though no muscles are being moved. The thoughts we think actually reshape our brains![5]

THOUGHTS INTO CAPTIVITY

Why must we bring every thought into captivity to Jesus? Because if we don't actively stop firing unhealthy neural circuits, those unhealthy thought patterns will not degrade and our characters will not be transformed in Christ's likeness. This is the meaning behind his famous reinterpretation of adultery: "You have heard that it was said, 'You shall not commit adultery.' But I tell you that anyone who looks at a woman lustfully has already committed adultery with her in his heart" (Mt 5:27-28). Jesus knew, of course, that if we continue to commit sin in our imaginations, those unhealthy circuits grow stronger and our characters cannot be healed.

One Bible writer says, in the old King James Version, "For as he thinketh in his heart, *so is* he" (Prov 23:7, emphasis mine). The decisions we make in our hearts determine which neural circuits get fired, either in action or imagination. But either way, it is the neural circuits the heart chooses that get activated and thus strengthened and retained. As mentioned in chapter 2, the neurological "heart" is the anterior cingulate cortex (ACC). It is the ACC that is the processing point between our judgment (DLPFC and OFC/VMPFC) and our emotions (limbic system). Ultimately, it is in the ACC that our choices are made.[6]

Why must we demolish every lie about God? Because when the ACC accepts such lies, unhealthy neural circuits get fired and grow stronger, the prefrontal cortex is damaged, love is impaired, and fear is inflamed. Ultimately, holding to lies about God prevents him from restoring his image within us. But when we accept the truth and worship the God of love, the PFC—including the ACC—grows healthier and fear is overcome.

A SCARY PICTURE OF GOD

Is God like the enemy alleges, or is God like Jesus revealed him to be? This is the question we all must answer. Our eternal salvation depends on which conclusion we draw. And we have another standard against which to test our theories. Is God a power monger, a being of stern justice who must use his power to inflict penalties? Does God say, "All I want is your love, but if you don't love me I will burn you in hell and torture you until you die?" Is God a being who requires appeasement? Is he a being who must be bought off by the blood of his son so he won't kill us? (This is not to say that the unrepentant won't die in the end; they will. But the *reason* they die is not that God is forced to torture and execute. Later we will explore why they die.)

In *Rediscovering the Scandal of the Cross,* Joel Green and Mark Baker recognize that the Bible provides no basis for such a fear-inducing God-construct. "Whatever meaning atonement might have, it would be a grave error to imagine that it focused on assuaging God's anger or winning God's merciful attention. . . . The Scripture as a whole provides no ground for a portrait of an angry God needing to be appeased in atoning sacrifice."[7]

There are only two gods to be worshiped: a God of love, as revealed in Jesus, or a god that is something other than love—a being who requires some action be taken in order to merit his mercy, forgiveness and grace. In every false religion of the world, the central fallacy is a distorted picture of God. He is either a being who is too busy to care, who is detached and disinterested, or who is a cruel tyrant of absolute power that must be appeased. Brain research has demonstrated that the kind of God you worship changes your brain. Only the worship of the God of love brings healing. Holding to lies obstructs the healing process.

As the world approaches the final consummation, what will the last contest with evil be over? What is the culmination of events as the Bible predicts? It will be a conflict over worship, over two systems, over two pictures of God. On the one hand is the beast's system, which violates liberty—no one may buy or sell except him who has the mark of the beast (Rev 13:17); or God's system of love—"No one has greater love than this, to lay down one's life for one's friends" (Jn 15:13 NRSV). The world is being pushed headlong toward this final confrontation when every person will have to choose: violate liberty, or love God and others supremely.

And what is the result of worshiping a deity who does not value freedom? What is the consequence to believing in a supreme being who will use his power to destroy, one who must be appeased in order to forgive? Such beliefs violate the law of liberty and, just as in human relationships, the outcome is predictable: love is destroyed, rebellion instilled, individuality eroded and, as we have seen, the prefrontal cortex is damaged.[8]

Jesus said at the end of time the love of most will grow cold (Mt 24:12). Why? Because of wickedness. And as Paul states in Romans 1:18-31, wickedness is the result of rejecting the truth about God. Rejecting the knowledge of God always leads away from God's methods. Thus religious people can worship a god who coerces and controls. And love is destroyed when liberty is abused. Brain imaging has documented the phenomenon that, when we worship a vengeful god who abuses freedom, when we anticipate the return of a punishing god, our fear circuits grow stronger and our prefrontal cortexes are damaged—again, in the brain region where we experience love, empathy and selflessness. Paul said that in the last day some will have a *form* of godliness but deny its power (2 Tim 3:5). Paul is not talking about the agnostics and atheists. He is speaking of people who claim to believe in God, but deny the truth about him—about his character of love.[9]

When we have a form of godliness but worship a god who is like Satan alleges, love is destroyed, fear is increased and, over time, we become shadow people—people like Joe and Lynda, who have lost or are losing their ability to reason, people who worship out of fear of punishment, people who become unthinking empty shells and are afraid to have an independent thought. One example is the notion that faith only means, "God said it, I believe it, and that settles it." But faith does not mean that we don't ask any questions at all, that we take faith on faith. That type of "blind faith," far from being a virtue in itself, causes us to become people who rigidly cling to rules, rituals and ceremonies without understanding what they mean, and then criticizing those who practice different rituals. You see, "faith" in an abusive god causes us to become like the abusive god we serve and use our power to control others, dominate others and coerce others into our way of living.

POLITICAL ORIENTATION AND THE BRAIN

A fascinating study recently revealed differences in brain structure correlate with political orientation. The study demonstrated that greater conservatism was associated with increased gray matter volume in the right amygdala, whereas greater liberalism was associated with increased gray matter volume in the anterior cingulate cortex (ACC). These results were replicated in an independent sample of additional subjects. The study authors could not determine if these brain differences caused the varied political attitudes or were a result of those attitudes.[10]

Remember that the amygdala is where we experience fear, whereas the ACC is where we experience compassion, empathy and concern for others. While the study authors could not determine if the brain differences they noted were caused by the various political leanings or a result of those beliefs, it is my hypothesis that the differences were reinforced if not caused by the political persuasion. In fact, based on plasticity studies (studies on how neural circuits that fire together expand and grow stronger) on Newberg's research showing that meditation twelve minutes per day results in measurable growth in the ACC, and on brain changes due to occupation (such as increased gray matter volume in London cab drivers in the part of the brain that deals with orientation in space),[11] I think that the divergent political attitudes contribute to the brain differences seen between liberals and conservatives.

If I am right, this is incredibly good news and fits well with God's promise to give us new hearts, heal our minds and re-create us within. It also fits with the recorded histories of various biblical figures. Saul of Tarsus, by any measure, was a very conservative individual. He was legalistic, rigid and intolerant, and he practiced methods of coercion. He had no problem using the power of the state to promote his religious beliefs. But after his conversion, Saul—the apostle Paul—was gracious, liberal in charity, self-sacrificing, patient, and ultimately willing to give his life for others. Such a drastic change would most certainly require the activation of different brain circuits. We could hypothesize that preconversion Saul had a very developed amygdala and an underdeveloped ACC, but then we would have to also allow that in the converted Paul the reverse was true. What this suggests is that, when we experience a change in belief about God and trust him, a new motive springs into the heart and new neural circuits fire resulting in positive brain changes.

When we worship distorted characterizations of God, love is destroyed and individuality is eroded. Or, sadly, many people who continue to think and reason for themselves, having never heard an alternative view of God (one of love), reject the idea of God altogether and become agnostics or athcists.

NOT BY MIGHT

God will not win this war for our hearts and restore us to love by the use of might and power. "'Not by might nor by power, but by my Spirit,' says the LORD Almighty" (Zech 4:6). As we discovered above, real change only occurs when it happens in the mind, when the thoughts change, thus changing the brain.

We can and sometimes must lock criminals in jail to "control" behavior, but we cannot control their imaginations. And if the thoughts do not change, the brain does not change, and therefore, the character does not change. God has the power to enforce behavior modification, but God cannot force a thought to alter course without destroying the individual and creating robots. Love cannot be commanded. Therefore, God cannot be telling us, "Love me or I'll kill you. Love me or I will be forced to torture you in hell forever." All such concepts—when compared to the constant, when compared to our standard, when compared to the laws of love and liberty—are revealed to be lies.

This was initially very hard for me to grasp. For much of my life I didn't understand and ran from the God of the Old Testament. I used to be confused because of all the times in the Bible where God did use might and power: the flood; Sodom and Gomorrah; the firstborn of Egypt; 185,000 Assyrians; the platoons that came to arrest Elijah; Korah, Dathan and Abirum; Uzzah, Nadab and Abihu. There are numerous instances in the Bible where God used his power to put people to rest in the grave. I had been taught this was proof that God does kill, that God does lose his patience, that God does get mad and, at some point, lash out to destroy his children.

As I look back at that time in my life, it was like gazing at the world through my grandmother's glasses. As a child I remember sitting next to grandma in church and putting on her glasses, as thick as Coke-bottle bottoms. The world went blurry. Everything was out of focus. I could no longer tell what I was looking at.

Likewise, I had examined God's Word through the lenses of distortion, tradition and misunderstanding, not comprehending what I was reading. I had too many lies in my mind. I needed a new set of glasses. I needed Jesus! I had failed to let Jesus be the lens through which I understood Scripture. I needed the living Word to define the written Word. I needed to become Jesus' friend and let him teach me. It was when I saw God's character of love, as revealed in Jesus, that the Bible finally came into focus.

When I looked to Jesus, I discovered something mind-boggling. Jesus—God in human flesh—did not describe death like we do. "When Jesus entered the synagogue leader's house and saw the noisy crowd and people playing pipes, he said, 'Go away. The girl is not dead but asleep.' But they laughed at him" (Mt 9:23-24). Why did they laugh at him? Because from their human perspective, the girl was dead.

Was Jesus lying when he said, "The girl is not dead but asleep"? Was he trying to mislead or deceive, to create misunderstanding and darken their minds? Or was he simply trying to be the light that enlightens all men? Was Jesus gently attempting to open their minds, even when all they could do was laugh? When compared to the principles of truth and openness that Jesus advocated, I couldn't believe Jesus would do anything deceptive, therefore, I concluded Jesus was trying to reveal greater truth.

MORE EVIDENCE

I searched for more evidence in another story of Christ coming face to face with someone who had died. "After he [Jesus] had said this, he went on to tell them, 'Our friend Lazarus has fallen asleep; but I am going there to wake him up.' His disciples replied, 'Lord, if he sleeps, he will get better.' Jesus had been speaking of his death, but his disciples thought he meant natural sleep. So then he told them plainly, 'Lazarus is dead'" (Jn 11:11-14). Again I asked myself, was Jesus lying? Was he trying to trick the disciples? Was he trying to create confusion, or was he attempting to open their minds to truth? I realized that Jesus was revealing heavenly light and that, if I wanted my mind to heal, I had to embrace it. With this new understanding in mind, I reexamined all those Old Testament stories that had troubled me for so long.

I asked myself, *If I allow Jesus to be my lens, if I allow God in human form to be the source of my definition of death, then has God killed anyone?* I was blown away as I realized that God has put millions of his children to sleep in the grave, but since that is not what God defines as death, then God has killed no one. In the mind of God, sleep and death are not the same. They serve very different purposes.

For instance, the Bible does not teach that the wages of sin is *sleep* or that sin, when it is full grown, brings forth *sleep* (Rom 6:23; Jas 1:15). In the language of God, sleep is temporary, death is permanent. Power down a computer, unplug the power cord and remove the battery, and it will "sleep," waiting to be energized, to "awaken," with all its data perfectly intact. But toss the computer in a hot fire and melt it, and then it will be destroyed, no awakening for that computer (unless there was a hard-drive backup waiting to be downloaded into a new machine). Was Jesus suggesting that what we call death is actually like a computer having its energy source removed, but that, to God, death is when the intelligent being is eternally destroyed?[12]

If so, then according to God, no one has yet died, but all sleep, waiting to be awakened by him at either the resurrection of life or the resurrection of damnation (Dan 12:13; Jn 5:29; 1 Thess 4:13). But this concept raised more questions. Why would God use his power to put people in the grave, to "power them down"?

As I was pondering this, I stumbled onto an amazing realization: God has not acted to put his children in the grave, as he did before Christ came, since Christ's resurrection. Why? Has the world, since the time of Christ, become a more loving, kind and gracious place? Has evil disappeared? Are there no longer problems of hedonism, idolatry, violence or abuse equal to what transpired prior to Christ's arrival on earth?

I thought of human history since Christ's resurrection: Nero, Stalin, Hitler, Amin, cannibalism, the worship of Kali the Hindu goddess of death, World War I, World War II, Rwanda, Bosnia. . . . I realized that evil has continued unabated after the cross, just as it did prior to it. But despite all this abuse, I didn't find God intervening as he did before the cross, and I wondered why.

I understood that whatever the reason for God's action, it could not be as I had been taught since childhood—that God inflicted punishment for sin. If punishment were the reason, then he would still be doling it out, since wickedness has in no way diminished. I realized, even using the logic of those who believe God does inflict punishment for sin, that he would never inflict it before judgment. And since the judgment hasn't yet happened, then his actions in the past were not for the purpose of punishing. Then why, if not to punish, did God put so many people to rest in the grave during Old Testament times? Why do we see such a drastic difference pre- and post-cross?

Then it struck me. Humanity had severed the circle of love and was plummeting toward eternal death, a permanent, irreversible death. But God loved too much to let go. A Savior was promised, One who would reconnect the world to God's circle of love. God had to keep open the channel for Jesus to come, and Satan, knowing full well the eternal consequences of that coming, fought furiously to obstruct him. Prior to the cross, God intervened to keep open the avenue for our Savior to make that journey from the courts of heaven to the manger in Bethlehem. But, once Jesus completed his mission on earth, God no longer needed to work in this way. The circle of love had been rejoined.

SON OF SALVATION

Once Adam sinned, the only way God could save humanity was by sending his Son. Right there in Eden, God promised a Savior—the offspring to crush the serpent's head (Gen 3:15). Satan knew that his hold on this world was not secure, that Jesus was coming to rescue us, to break the bonds of Satan's kingdom, to set us free. Therefore, he immediately began contending, with all his evil ability, to prevent Jesus from coming and to close the avenue through which the Messiah would arrive. How? By enticing every human being to close their heart to God, such that no woman would voluntarily become the mother of Jesus.

I realized when God destroyed the world with a flood, there was only one righteous man left on the earth. Only one. The avenue through which Christ would appear was about to close. But Love would not let go. God intervened by allowing millions of his unruly children to rest in the grave, not as a punishment, but in order to save the planet, in order to keep his connection with us, in order to keep that channel open. How hard that must have been for God!

Imagine you have ten children: five are over the age of twenty and five are under the age of seven. The older children are rebellious, abusers, molesters, drug addicts, murderers and are bent on molesting and murdering your five younger children. Every attempt on your part to bring your older children to repentance is met with contempt and attacks against you. If you had the ability to put those older children in cryogenic storage—not to kill them, just power them down, put them in suspended animation long enough for your younger children to grow up safely—and then reanimate your unruly older children, would you do it? Would you put your older children in "time out," literally taking them out of time, until your younger children were mature; then thaw the older ones out to finish their lives? Isn't that what God was doing in the Old Testament? God intervened in love, but Satan twisted God's action into an act of vengeance, creating terrifying views of God, leading us to be afraid of God, because lies believed break the circle of love and trust, inflame the limbic system and impair the prefrontal cortex's function. And love cannot flow where lies about God abound.

I looked to the cross for the truth of how God treats sinners and realized Jesus was not a helpless victim like the two thieves. All power had been given to him (Jn 13:3). He was the Creator, the King of heaven and earth. As I contemplated this, I remembered the old television programs I Dream of Jeannie and Bewitched, and I realized Jesus didn't have to blink his eyes or twitch his nose to make things happen. Jesus only had to think, Be gone, and the entire mob would have been wiped out. Imagine, in the face of such torture on the cross, he did not even have the thought, "I wish you were gone."

What incredible love that, in the midst of horrible abuse, Christ never had a single thought to harm his attackers or to save himself! I remembered the old saying, "Power corrupts and absolute power corrupts absolutely" and knew it was not so with Jesus. He proved, beyond any doubt, that he is safe with all power because he will never use his power in self-interest. What an awesome God! He'd rather let his creatures abuse and kill him than use his power to stop them. What freedom, what liberty we have with God. Truly, worthy, worthy, worthy is the Lamb who was slain. He is worthy to have all power because he has proven he is safe with all power.

Love can only exist in an atmosphere of freedom. God is love, and what he wants can only be obtained through the use of his methods: truth, presented in love, leaving others free.

The breach in love began when lies about God replaced the truth. God's healing remedy commences with the truth. "Then you will know the truth, and the truth will set you free" (Jn 8:32).

The Battle Between the Conflicting Views About God

5

Love Strikes Back

Love has nothing to do
with what you are expecting to get;
it's what you are expected to give
—which is everything.

ANONYMOUS

SHE WAS ONLY NINETEEN AND SUFFERING, in terrible pain, when I met her. Her body was broken, but she was lucky to be alive. Sam, short for Samantha, was the talk of the hospital, a miracle of sorts. She had joined the U.S. Army right after high school and enlisted for Special Forces training and military jump school at Fort Bragg.

Soon after completing basic training, she arrived at Fort Bragg for the grueling preparation of a paratrooper. She learned how to pack her own chute, properly load her equipment and safely exit a plane. She was taught how to cut away a faulty chute and deploy her reserve in case of emergency. She practiced the proper way to land, crumple and roll. She completed all of her training jumps without any difficulty and was proud of her accomplishment when graduation day finally arrived.

The families of the graduates were invited to a ceremony unlike any other in the country. Graduates at Fort Bragg don't walk down the aisle in robe and mortar board with an orchestra playing "Pomp and Circumstance," but instead, they float down by parachute in full combat dress to the roar of Hercules C-130s flying by. With the stands full of excited family members, the planes began to pass overhead and chute after chute opened, decorating the sky with little green soldiers dancing in the wind. The graduates landed on the parade field in front of the bleachers from where their families watched.

Suddenly, a gasp rose from the audience as one chute failed to open. With all eyes riveted to the soldier streaming through the sky, the anxious crowd watched as the tangled chute was cut away and the emergency chute was deployed. But then screams filled the parade ground as the emergency chute also tangled and failed to open. Sam's parents had no idea that she was the soldier whose chute had failed to deploy. Mom and Dad watched in stunned silence, praying for the unknown soldier whom they would later learn was their daughter.

Sam followed her training; when she hit the ground, she crumpled and rolled. The force of the impact broke both legs, her pelvis and caused some damage to her sacral spine. But, amazingly, she survived.

I remember the buzz around the hospital. "What a miracle; God must really have a purpose for her life," said one nurse. But she was quickly challenged by another who said, "If God were going to perform a miracle, why didn't he just have the parachute work? No, I wonder what she did to offend God that he would do this to her."

I thought about Sam and why she got injured. Did the "good" God intervene to save her? Did the "bad" god intervene to punish her? Did the "ugly" god not care?

NATURAL LAW

I knew that if Sam happened to receive the chute she herself had packed, her parents wouldn't hate her for failing to pack her chute correctly. That's when it struck me: God doesn't hate humankind for falling into sin. What Sam's parents hated was that Sam had jumped out of a plane with a parachute that didn't work. Why? Because it resulted in pain and suffering to the one they loved.

Again, assuming Sam received the chute she packed, no one had to inflict punishment on her for failing to pack it correctly. Even though the Army had given Sam explicit instructions on how to pack a chute, if she failed to comply with those rules, the government did not have to inflict punishment on her in order to be just. Instead, the government intervened to stop what justly should occur when one jumps from an airplane without a working parachute. As soon as she hit the ground, the same government that told her how to avoid damage bent its resources on healing the damage done.

Ground emergency responders, ambulances, medics, doctors, nurses, physical therapists—all the governmental resources necessary to save and heal Sam—were immediately mobilized. Even before she slammed into the ground, the government's interventions began. Emergency responders were already moving to meet her at the point of impact.

Thinking about this modern scene, I imagined the shrieks of horror resounding throughout heaven as the angels watched Adam and Eve believe the lies of the serpent, partake of the fruit and plummet toward their eternal demise. But God was already moving, before they landed in sin, to meet their urgent need. Jesus, the "Lamb who was slain from the creation of the world" (Rev 13:8) was already there to catch them in his arms of love.

Every agency in God's government leapt into action in order to heal and save, not only Adam and Eve, but you and me as well. Lies believed broke the circle of love and trust. But, praise be to God,

Love would not let go. Love struck back. Jesus stepped in. The human race—of which we are all members—would be saved!

LOVE'S INTERCESSION

Love could not abandon us. God could not turn his back on us. He would rather die than let us go. Even though lies were believed, even though the human brain was no longer loving but fearful and selfish, even though death was stalking humanity, God was instantly pouring himself out to save and heal.

As soon as our first parents believed lies about God, broke the circle of love and trust, and corrupted themselves with the me-first principle, Love reached down from heaven and began intercession. God stepped in; he put himself between us and sin's cancerous assault. He intervenes to cure humanity, to save us from eternal death.

GOD INTERCEDES IN THREE WAYS:

1. He opposes the principalities and powers of darkness by holding evil forces in check. The Bible says he sends his angels to restrain the four winds (Rev 7:1) and places a hedge of protection around his people, deterring satanic agencies (2 Kings 6:17; Job 1:10; Ps 91:11).

2. God also intercedes in our hearts and minds. He sends his Spirit to work in our brains to enlighten with truth, to convict, to draw, to woo, to place a desire for good—a longing for love into our hearts (Gen 3:15; Jn 16:8). Ever since the fall of Adam and Eve, Love has been warring with evil, obstructing its deadly intent while simultaneously fighting to eradicate the infection of fear and selfishness from the human heart.

3. Jesus interceded in the course of sinfulness itself. He became sin for us (2 Cor 5:21). He took on himself our terminal condition in order to conquer, overcome and cure. "Surely he took up our infirmities and carried our sorrows" (Is 53:4 NIV 1984). Yes, Jesus became one of us in order to reverse all the damage

sin has done to his creation and to restore us, his children, back to unity with God. Jesus came to crush the serpent's head (Gen 3:15) — to destroy Satan and eradicate the sin infection from this world (Heb 2:14).

Because of God's intercession, there are now two antagonistic principles at war on planet Earth — love and survival of the fittest. God's principle of love was summed up by Jesus laying down his life for us (Jn 15:13). This means, "I love you so much that I will do whatever I have to for your health, welfare and good, including if necessary, giving my life that you might live." Such godly love is at war with the survival-of-the-fittest principle, which says, "I love myself so much I will do whatever I have to in order to protect, advance and exalt myself including, if necessary, killing you that I might live." Give my life that you might live, or kill you that I might live. These are the two principles at war in each of our hearts.

KNOWING THE TRUTH

God is working, via his Spirit, to enlighten, heal and restore. Jesus said, "You will know the truth, and the truth will set you free" (Jn 8:32).

Truth enters the mind through the circuits of the prefrontal cortex. But the enemy not only tries to confuse our thinking with lies, he also inflames our limbic systems. "When tempted, no one should say, 'God is tempting me.' For God cannot be tempted by evil, nor does he tempt anyone; but each person is tempted when they are dragged away by their own evil desire and enticed. Then, after desire has conceived, it gives birth to sin; and sin, when it is full-grown, gives birth to death" (Jas 1:13-15). Our evil desires arise from our limbic systems, our own centers of emotion and desire.

God is constantly working to heal and restore perfect love in our hearts, using only his methods of truth, love and freedom. Satan, the polar opposite of love, is working to destroy. The father of lies twists, distorts and misrepresents all God's interventions of love because, as we've learned, lies believed break the circle of love and trust and keep us afraid of God. When we respond to God's love and practice his methods, our higher brain regions grow stronger. But when we choose selfishness, our limbic systems grow stronger, guilt increases and prefrontal-cortex function is impaired. It is only by coming back into a trusting relationship with God that our brains can be healed and our characters purified.

A REMOTE VILLAGE

Imagine a remote village in Africa. No modern Westerner has ever set foot there. The natives live off the land, using the same ancient methods and tools as their forefathers used for the last thousand years. They know nothing of modern science, technology or medicine.

One day a group of medical missionaries comes to this village to provide whatever health care might be needed. The day they arrive they meet a child writhing in pain near the edge of the encampment. Examining the child, they quickly diagnose acute appendicitis. Without emergency surgery he will die.

Fortunately, the medical missionaries have a mobile surgical suite and all the necessary equipment to perform this life-saving operation. They pick up the child, kicking and screaming, and begin the emergency intervention. As the medical team works furiously to save the child's life, three other children watch intensely from a nearby hiding place. The medical personnel hold the child while a nurse sticks a needle in his arm and infuses fluids. The terrified patient squirms violently until medicine is injected and he quickly becomes unresponsive. The three children are frightened as they watch a masked man take a sharp knife and cut open their friend's abdomen. In terror they run to their village, screaming that invaders are coming to capture them, put them on a table and carve them up like pigs.

The entire village is aroused. The children, the elderly, the weak and the frightened quickly begin an evacuation, running from this terrible threat. The warriors begin devising plans to fight against this hostile invader. When the medical missionaries finally approach the village, they are attacked and driven away. No one in that community is going to be foolish enough to let these barbarians near.

What could the medical team do to engender trust? If they had called in soldiers and taken the village by force, would trust be restored? If only the missionaries had a member of that tribe, someone who knew the people and spoke their language, to go ahead of them and tell the villagers the truth. If only someone from that health-care team could be born into that village, grow up among them, and reveal they were friends and not enemies.

This is how it is with God and the human race ever since our first parents broke the circle of love and trust. We are sick and dying. God has been working to save and heal, to restore us to trust so we will let him cure us. But our darkened minds, like those of the villagers, have all too often misunderstood what God is trying to do. We have viewed God as terrifying or hostile and, as a result, have rejected his messengers, attacked his prophets and driven away his representatives. "Darkness covers the earth and thick darkness is over the peoples" (Is 60:2). Therefore, God sent us his Son, the "true light, which enlightens everyone" (Jn 1:9 NRSV) to reveal God's true character in order to win us back to trust, to connect us back to the circle of love. But sadly, though "the light shines in the darkness, . . . the darkness has not understood it" (Jn 1:5 NIV 1984). Until we understand the light—the truth about God as revealed in Jesus— our minds cannot be healed. Why? Because lies believed inflame the limbic system and damage the prefrontal cortex, obstructing the flow of love in our being. The truth, on the other hand, destroys lies, restores trust and, as we build that trust relationship with God, his lifesaving love begins to flow through us again. It is that love flowing through us that heals the brain and transforms the soul.

The first step in the healing process is coming to the truth about God.

THE BATTLE IN THE CONVERTED BRAIN

It is truth about God that destroys lies and wins us back to trust. In trust we open our hearts and experience God's love, which overcome fear and enable us to give rather than constantly seek to get. This is conversion, the experience of a fundamental switch in the primary motive of the heart—from our inherent survival-of-the-fittest selfishness to other-centered love.

Although we can experience conversion in a moment (the thief on the cross next to Christ, Saul on the road to Damascus), God's healing transformation of our lives occurs gradually, steadily, progressively. It takes time for unhealthy neural circuits to degrade and healthy ones to form.

Consider being infected with anthrax. Without treatment, you will die. The infection has already caused significant damage by the time you go to the doctor. The doctor provides an antibiotic that will cure your condition, but you have to trust the doctor and follow his treatment plan. The moment you take your first dose of antibiotic, you have left the path of death and entered life. This would be analogous to conversion. But will all of your symptoms be resolved that day? Or will there be a gradual healing process?

Likewise, we were all born dead in trespasses and sin—a terminal condition of selfishness (Ps 51:5; Eph 2:1). But when we see the truth about God, we enter at conversion into a trust relationship with Jesus Christ and accept his treatment for our lives; we leave the path of death and enter into eternal life. It is in this saving relationship that God's healing power begins working in our lives. However, until Christ returns, the healing of our minds, the transformation of our characters, the rewiring of our brains is an ongoing battle as old neural circuits are degraded and healthy pathways are formed.

This is what Paul was describing in Romans 7. I have paraphrased what I believe Paul is saying, inserting some insights regarding brain physiology:

What shall we say then? Is the written law evil and selfish because it increases the amount of evil and selfishness we see? Absolutely not! For I would not have known what evil and selfishness look like if it wasn't for the diagnostic efficacy of the written law. I would not have realized that coveting was evil and selfish if the commandment didn't say, "Don't covet." But selfishness, taking advantage of the fact that the written law is only a diagnostic instrument and not a remedy, magnified every covetous desire within me. For apart from the diagnostic ability of the written law, sin is unrecognizable. Once I thought I was healthy and free from the infection of distrust, fear and selfishness, but then the commandment examined me, exposed how utterly infected I was and diagnosed me as terminal. I discovered that the very commandment given only to diagnose my condition I had unwittingly attempted to use as a cure, and thus my condition only worsened. For selfishness, taking advantage of the fact that the commandment could only diagnose and not cure, deceived me into thinking I could be cured by working to keep the commandments, but instead my terminal state only worsened. So understand this: the written law diagnoses perfectly, and the commandment is the standard of what is right and good, set apart by God, to reveal what is evil and destructive.

Did the law, which did good by diagnosing what was wrong with me, become the source of my terminal condition? Of course not! It only exposed what was already in me so that I could recognize how totally decayed, putrid and near death I was, so that through the lens of the commandment I might become utterly disgusted with evil and selfishness and long for a cure.

We know that the written law is consistent, reliable and reasonable; but I am inconsistent, unreliable and unreasonable, because the infection of distrust, fear and selfishness has warped my mind and damaged my thinking. I am frustrated with what I do. For having been restored to trust, I want to do what is in harmony with God and his methods of love; but I find that even though I trust God, old habits, conditioned responses, preconceived ideas and other remnants of the devastation caused by distrust and selfishness are not yet fully removed. And if I find an old habit causing me to behave in ways that I now find detestable, I affirm that the written law is a very helpful tool for revealing residual damage in need of healing. What is happening is this: In my prefrontal cortex I have come to trust God and desire to do his will, but old habits and conditioned responses, which arise from unhealthy neural circuits that fire my limbic system, occur almost reflexively in certain situations. These unhealthy neural circuits have not yet been totally eliminated and thus cause me do to things I do not want to do. I know my mind used to be completely infected with distrust, fear and selfishness, which totally perverted all my desires and faculties, so that even when distrust had been eradicated and trust had been restored, the damage caused by years of distrustful and selfish behavior has not yet been fully healed. So I find, at times, I have the desire to do what is right, but my prefrontal cortex is not fully healed, thus I do not yet have the ability to carry out the desire. For the old habits and conditioned responses from unhealthy neural circuits that activate my limbic system are not the good I want to do; no, they are remnants of my selfish unconverted mind. So if I find myself doing what I no longer desire to do, it is not I, but vestiges of old habits and conditioned responses that have yet to be removed, and through God's grace will soon be removed.

So, I find this reality at work: When I want to do good, old selfish habits and residual feelings of fear are right there with me. For in my prefrontal cortex I rejoice in God's methods and principles; but I recognize I remain damaged from years of being infected with distrust and practicing Satan's methods, so that even though the infection of distrust has been removed, the old habits of fear and self-promotion tempt me from within. What a damaged and corrupt man I am! Who will deliver and heal me from a brain and body so diseased and deformed? Praise be to God—for he has provided the healing solution through Jesus Christ our Lord! So then, I find that in my prefrontal cortex I am now renewed with trust for God and love of his methods, but my entire brain and body remain damaged by years of self-indulgent behavior.

At long last, I could see it so clearly: lies believed break the circle of love and trust. Without love and trust, fear and selfishness consume the mind. Our brains are damaged and filled with every kind of twisted and distorted idea about God, frantically seeking relief, but only sinking into deeper confusion. It is only when the good news about God removes the distorted and twisted views of him that our minds can heal.

6

Engaging the Battle

The inevitability of the death of Jesus
does not stem from God's need but from humanity's.
There are only two roles to play in the tale of divine and
human relationships, persecutor or persecuted.
God can cause suffering or God can suffer.
God in Christ chose the latter.

MICHAEL HARDIN

SAVANNAH WAS FIFTEEN WITH RED HAIR and aqua green eyes. When she smiled, an intoxicating energy beamed from her like light from the sun. But this day Savannah wasn't smiling; her face was somber, the sun had gone out. She barely made eye contact and her shoulders drooped, burdened with guilt and self-loathing. She sat almost motionless, staring at her hands.

Her parents had brought her to see me because Savannah had not been herself lately. About three weeks prior they had noticed a change. Her normal sparkle and vibrancy had become clouded over with a near impenetrable gloom. Her appetite had waned as well as her weight; she had dropped ten pounds in three weeks. She had stopped talking on her cell phone or texting her friends. She had lost interest in life and isolated herself from her family, preferring the seclusion of her bed. Her parents were rightly concerned and began to fear Savannah might be suicidal.

The girl was very guarded. She didn't want to see a psychiatrist. She didn't want to be in my office. This made helping her all the more difficult.

After her parents left the room I said quietly, "Savannah, what's going on that your parents brought you to see me?"

Silence.

"Did you want to come here today?"

Without looking up she said, "Why can't they just leave me alone?"

"Who?"

"Everyone. Why can't everyone just leave me alone?"

"Your parents love you too much to do nothing when they see you hurting."

There was no verbal response, but tears began to form in her eyes; I could see she did care. I waited briefly and then asked, "Would you prefer to have parents who don't care about you, parents who would leave you alone when they see you in pain?"

She continued to stare at her hands. I prayed silently, *Lord, give me wisdom to help her. Send your Spirit to soften her heart, strengthen and comfort her, and your angels to drive back any evil forces.*

"That's all I deserve," she whispered as she began to weep.

"What's all you deserve?"

"I don't deserve parents who care."

"Why do you think you don't deserve your parents who love and care for you?" I waited, and gently asked, "Savannah, what happened?"

"I did it." She blurted.

"Did what?"

"It!" She looked at me, her eyes pleading as if to add, *Please don't make me say it.*

I said it for her: "You had sex?"

She cried as she nodded.

Slowly, painfully, she told me what had happened. After school three weeks earlier she decided to go riding around with two guys she didn't know all that well. At first it was fun, listening to music, complaining about school and talking about other kids. But then it got uncomfortable.

While one young man was driving, the other began to make advances. Savannah said she didn't intend to have sex with him but didn't know what to do. She didn't want the guys to be mad at her, didn't want them to dislike her, so she didn't say no. She squirmed a little, tried to turn away a little, but as the boy continued his verbal pressure, she succumbed to his exploitation. Savannah's prefrontal cortex wanted to say no, but the fear and insecurity from the amygdala was paralyzing her good judgment.

By now she was crying hard, not looking at me, her face buried in her hands. Her body language exuded shame, guilt and fear—fear of rejection, fear of never being loved, fear of ruining her life. So I said, "How do you feel?"

"Horrible! Worthless, no good!"

"Are you afraid you have ruined your life?"

She nodded, still not looking up.

Given her reaction I wondered if she held a punitive view of God, so I asked, "Are you afraid you have sinned so bad that God can never love you again; that you are too dirty, too awful and too bad for God to forgive? Are you afraid *God* is mad at you?"

Instantly, before the words had finished leaving my mouth she looked at me, a terrible fear and panic on her face. With a desperate pleading in her eyes, she sobbed, "How could he? I had sex. I lost my virginity. How could anyone ever love me again?"

Fear was tormenting her soul—fear of rejection, fear of ruin, fear of condemnation, fear of embarrassment. It was consuming her thoughts, stealing her joy. I knew that before she could get well, that terrible fear must abate. But she believed lies about herself and lies about God, and lies obstruct the flow of healing love. In fact, the lies she believed caused her prefrontal cortex to further inflame her limbic system rather than calm it. She needed to experience the truth, spoken in love.

I gave her some time to calm down, then asked, "Are you tired of hurting? Are you tired of the guilt? Are you tired of being miserable? Would you like to heal, like to find peace and happiness again?"

"Oh, yes!" She said, but her eyes questioned, *Is it possible?*

"Do you remember the story of Adam's fall?"

She nodded.

"After Adam sinned and was hiding in the Garden," I told her, "God gently called out to him. God knew where Adam was, of course, but notice how gentle God is. He called out to Adam not wanting to frighten him further than he already was. 'Adam, where are you?' God said."

I opened my Bible and read Adam's reply, "I heard you in the garden, and I was afraid because I was naked; so I hid." Then I asked Savannah to notice God's amazing reply, "Who told you that you were naked?" (See Gen 3:9-11.)

"Think it through," I said softly. "In the Garden, what were the possible answers to God's question? How many people were around to tell Adam he was naked? So what is the point of God's question? When God asked, 'Who told you that you are naked?' God is saying, 'Adam, my son, I am not the one pointing out your nakedness. You didn't hear me say you were naked. Adam, it's your own conscience that is condemning you, not me. You're feeling so bad because your brain is no longer in balance, like I designed it to be. I love you and I am here to save you!'"

Savannah's eyes grew wide with hope. Her mind was working. Could it be true?

I continued, "Do you remember the story of the woman caught in adultery?"

She nodded, this time a little quicker.

"After Jesus had dispatched the crowd and only he and this woman remained, notice what he said regarding her accusers. 'Where are they? Has no one condemned you?' [Jn 8:10]. Who were the only people in this conversation? Jesus and the woman. And what is the point of Jesus' question? He was saying, 'Hey, I am not the one condemning you. I know everything about you. I know what you were just involved in and you don't hear accusations coming from me. I love you! I'm here to save and heal you.' And just so there is no mistaking our understanding of this encounter, Jesus explicitly stated, 'Neither do I condemn you.' Then he added, 'Leave here renewed, live a life victorious over sin'" (Jn 8:11, my paraphrase).

"Savannah," I gently said, "God doesn't condemn you. He's not mad at you. God loves you. He wants to save and heal you. The condemnation is coming from your own conscience, not from God."

It was obvious in my young patient that she desperately wanted to believe that God wasn't condemning her, that God still loved her. I could see her heart was being drawn toward the truth, but she wasn't yet free. There were more distortions in her mind, more misunderstandings that needed purging, more truth needing to be understood. So I said, "I am so glad your conscience is hurting as badly as it is and causing you so much guilt."

She looked at me puzzled, wondering if I thought she deserved to suffer.

"Why would it be a good thing for you to feel pain when you touch a hot stove?" I asked.

"So I would pull back my hand."

"Exactly! So, by doing that, you would minimize any damage. And if you were sensitive enough, you might feel the heat before you actually touched the stove and never even get burned. Our consciences are sensitive to actions that will do much worse than burn our bodies.

Our consciences sense things that actually damage and destroy our hearts, our minds, our characters. And just like pain from touching a hot stove is designed to get us to pull back quickly in order to minimize damage, appropriate guilt is designed to get us to stop whatever we are doing that is damaging our characters, thereby minimizing the damage. And just like the pain after an injury motivates us to go to the doctor for treatment and healing, the guilt from sin is designed to get us to go to God for his treatment and eternal healing."

"So guilt isn't a bad thing?" she asked.

"Not at all, guilt is evidence that your heart and mind are sensitive to the working of the Holy Spirit. Guilt only becomes bad if, like pain, it never goes away. Think about it, after what you have gone through, are you more likely or less likely to give in to a guy's inappropriate advances?"

A tiny smile played at the corners of her mouth. "I'd kick his butt first!"

I laughed, "Absolutely!"

That was enough for one session. Savannah wiped away her tears and thanked me profusely as she left. But I knew there was much more work to do.

"God did not send his Son into the world to condemn the world, but to save the world through him" (Jn 3:17). God is reaching out with love and truth, but sadly our darkened minds and fearful hearts have not understood. Until we accept the truth about God, our minds cannot be healed. So love battles on.

7

Love Stands Firm

Our true identity is to love without fear
and insecurity. Our higher potential finds us
when we set our course in that direction.
The power of love and compassion
transforms insecurity.

DOC CHILDRE

WHEN I WAS SIX YEARS OLD I attended first grade in a small two-room Christian school in rural South Jersey. Grades one through five met in one room; six through eight met in another. One of the joys of recess was swinging on one of the three wood-seated swings in our small playground. When recess finally arrived, we children would race to the swings, eager to secure one of the few coveted seats. Those of us in first grade rarely got to swing, as the older children were much faster and almost always got there first.

As children often do, we began to think of other imaginative ways to have fun, and soon we discovered the excitement of running under the swing while an older student stood on the seat swinging powerfully back and forth. Lines quickly formed in front of each swing. One by one we would dash under the swing, timing our move just right to avoid getting hit. Soon it was my turn. I raced forward as fast as my first-grade legs would carry me, but my timing was off and *bam*, the swing smashed full force into my forehead, cutting a gash from which the blood started to pour.

I was knocked backward to the ground and began screaming in pain. My memory of the children shouting, the principal carrying me into the school and my mother driving me to the doctor are all vague and blurry. But I have a sharp and clear memory of being on the doctor's examining room table and seeing him coming at me with a needle that appeared, to my six-year-old eyes, to be five feet long. The closer he came, pushing that needle toward my forehead, it looked like he was going to stick it right in my eye.

I wanted to run, run away as fast as I possibly could, because I was afraid. But my mother held me tight. I tried to squirm free, I begged, I cried, but mother would not let go. She loved me too much. But my mother did more. She spoke words to me, loving words, encouraging words, reassuring me that she was there, that everything would be okay. While her reassurance didn't remove all fear from my six year-old mind, it did reduce it. Love and fear struggled against each other on a battlefield of pain.

My mother's love made me stand firm, for surely if she had not been there demonstrating that love, I would have run away. My limbic system was firing furiously, fear was increasing, and my child brain could not process the emotions I was experiencing and choose the healthy course. I wasn't mature enough to realize the importance of standing my ground. At age six, all I could think of was the pain. All I wanted was to avoid that needle. While, at age six, I couldn't understand why my mother would subject me to such pain, as an adult I am very thankful to my mother who held me tight, constraining me, even though it was painful, even though it was scary. Because of her love, I could heal.

What I realize now, which I did not appreciate then, is that letting fear take control (limbic system) only worsens the outcome. The wound would not have closed properly, infection may have set in, and if I didn't die, I would certainly have an ugly scar.

Fear and insecurity are so deeply woven into the fabric of my being that running seems so easy, almost right. I am still, far too often, like that little boy who needed mommy to hold me and make me stand my ground. Once injured, the healing path is always painful, and I don't like pain. My fear tempts me to run away—away from that apology, away from repentance, away from humbling myself, away from sharing my last meal with another. I want to run back to myself, my corner, my little world where I can drown out the truth I don't like. But I will never find peace if I keep running. I will never get well. Instead fear will only increase as the limbic system grows stronger.

Wounds are painful—whether physical, emotional or spiritual— and we are all wounded. It is love that heals our hearts. It is love that gives us strength to stand strong. It is love that overcomes fear.

LOVE STANDS STRONG

In February 2001, love pushed back against the darkness. Norina Bentzel, principal of the North Hopewell-Winterstown Elementary School in Red Lion, Pennsylvania, was just finishing a phone call when she saw a man enter the school. Thinking it might be one of the student's grandparents, she asked if she could help him. Suddenly, the man pulled out a machete and attacked Norina. He hit her shoulder and cut her hand. As he swung for her abdomen, she jumped back just in time to avoid a life-threatening wound.

The man turned and ran toward the classrooms where the children waited unsuspectingly. Norina screamed, "Call 911, Lockdown!" and ran to her office and hit the alarm, alerting the teachers to lock down their rooms. But she was too late to stop him from entering a kindergarten class of twenty-three students taught by fifty-three-year-old Linda Collier.

The crazed man came in swinging the machete. He cut one child's arm and just missed another child's neck, slicing off her ponytail as she pulled away. Linda began screaming, "Stop! What do you think you're doing? Stop hitting those children!" He turned on Linda and began swinging at her, gashing her hand. But the distraction was enough.

The children ran out of the room to the principal's office with the madman in hot pursuit. Norina quickly ushered the children into the room, and then, like a mother hen staring down a wolf, she stepped into the doorway between the attacker and his would-be victims. She stood there as the assailant rained blow after blow down upon her, but Norina would not move! He fractured her left forearm and nearly severed several of her fingers, but Norina stood her ground. Then, while he was pummeling her, Linda Collier and the school nurse jumped on the attacker's back and he collapsed, then surrendered. Thankfully both Norina and Linda survived.[1]

Love is not afraid. Love sacrifices self. Love does what is right.

LOVE STANDS UP

Ellen was distraught, desperate and overwhelmed. I could hear the anguish in her voice, see the agony on her face and feel the tension in the air. Her emotional cup was full. The pressure was too great; she couldn't contain it anymore. She had to find relief or her mind would burst.

As soon as I closed my office door she exploded. "I don't know what to do. I didn't know where to go. I don't know who to talk to. I can't believe I am here. I'm sorry, I shouldn't be here. I shouldn't have bothered you. I can't sleep. I can't think. What am I going to do? Can you help me?" The words poured out of her like water through a ruptured dam. She couldn't hold them back anymore.

"Ellen," I said gently, "You're safe here. Tell me, what's going on?"

"I shouldn't be here. I've never seen a psychiatrist before. I should be able to handle it."

"Handle what?"

She looked at me, silently sizing me up. Could she tell me? Could I handle it? Was she really safe here? Her eyes were uncertain as she glanced about the room. She was torn. I prayed silently, *Lord, send your angels here now. Create a haven of safety. Help Ellen find the words she needs. Give me wisdom to help.*

"It's my husband," she said. "I don't know what to do."

Aware of her struggle to open up, I started with some less emotionally charged questions, "How long have you been married?"

"Thirteen years."

"Is this your first marriage?"

"Yes."

"First for your husband as well?"

"Yes."

"Do you have children?"

"No."

"Tell me about your marriage."

"Our marriage has been great—at least I thought it was. I didn't think there were any problems. I love being a wife. I love making my husband happy. Whatever my husband wants I've always done."

Ellen told me they were Christians. She had been raised to believe the duty of a wife was to serve her husband, and she embraced this responsibility without question. She was proud to say that in her marriage she had never told her husband no. She had never denied one of his requests. She had never failed to meet one of his demands. She believed it was her Christian duty to submit herself to his leadership and direction, and she actually enjoyed living this role. Ellen believed that if you love your husband you do what he wants.

I wondered, *What does he want now?*

"Has submitting so completely to your husband's direction caused any problems for you?" I asked.

"Not until now."

"What happened?"

And finally, the truth poured out, "My husband turns forty in three weeks. He told me that, for his fortieth birthday," she paused, tears welling up in her eyes, searching for the words, "that for his fortieth birthday, he wants me to find another woman and bring her to our bed." She was crying, "I don't know what to do. I am supposed to submit to my husband. If you love your husband you're supposed to give him what he wants. I want to be a loving wife. I want to make him happy. I want to give him what he wants. But not this. I can't—not this. I don't know what to do. I don't want to disappoint him."

I saw the problem clearly. I knew what she needed (no, she didn't need a new husband). She needed to apply the law of love. Ellen's problem was not primarily her husband, even though he was part of the problem. Ellen's primary problem was her concept of God, her idea of what love is and how healthy relationships are designed to function. Ellen didn't yet know God's original design for humanity. She didn't know how healthy, godly love works. She had accepted a false concept, a distorted view. She didn't realize that real love does what is best for the other, not merely what the other person wants. The lie she believed impaired the function of her prefrontal cortex and, therefore, love could not flow, and her fear and anxiety could not be resolved.

I explored with her how genuine, Godlike love is the principle of beneficent, other-centered orientation. We want to do what will benefit others the most, from the perspective of their eternal best interest. This means we do not merely give what the other person wants but give what is actually best for them.

"Ellen," I said, "What is the 'loving' response from a parent when the child wants to watch TV instead of doing homework?"

"If she is thinking of what is best for the child, the answer is no TV."

"Exactly, and such action doesn't just provide the temporal benefits of getting good grades in school but also helps the child develop mature character, learn self-governance, self-discipline and the ability to sacrifice immediate rewards for long-term good. Such decision making is thinking of their eternal welfare and is genuinely loving in nature."

"But what happens if the parent is thinking of self, is afraid of how the child might respond, or if the parent needs the child's approval? What might that parent do?"

Ellen saw it clearly: "Give into the child's request so the parent could get what the parent wants—the child's approval."

"And might the parent then tell herself she is being selfless and giving and loving to the child? But this would be a lie. The loving course of action is to do what is best for the child, not what the child wants, even if the child gets upset for doing so."

"Love is the application of this principle to all relationships. If your husband has alcohol problems and asks you to buy him beer, what is the loving response? To do what he wants or lovingly say, 'Sweetheart, I love you. And because I love you I cannot assist in your self-destruction. I will do everything in my power for your good, your health and your welfare, but I cannot and I will not assist you in destroying yourself'?"

Ellen was trapped because she had accepted a lie about love. She believed love was sacrificing oneself to make another happy—to give another what he wanted—rather than sacrificing self to do what is actually best for the other person. Thus, whenever her husband said, "If you love me you will . . . ," she was conflicted. Her conscience convicted her of the wrongfulness of the request, but her idea of love told her that she should do what makes him happy. She was actually more concerned about keeping him contented with her than doing what was most loving. Her problem was her distorted idea of love, stemming from fear and insecurity.

RIGHT CHOICES

We all recognize the right choice for Ellen was to say no to her husband's lustful request. But why was that the right choice? Possible answers are, "Because giving in breaks God's commandment," or "Because it's just wrong," or "Because engaging in such activity desecrates my body—the spiritual temple of God." While all of these answers are true, if we apply the law of love to the question, what answer do we give? What is truly best for Ellen's husband? Is it in her husband's spiritual, eternal best interest for Ellen to say yes to his request? Of course not. Not only is it right in honoring God to say no, not only is it right in maintaining her own virtue, but if she loves her husband, if she is concerned with his eternal destiny, the answer is unequivocally, "No! I care too much about you, your character, your mind, your spiritual development and your eternal destiny to say yes. Such an act would damage you. It would sear your conscience, warp your character and damage your soul. I can't go along with that."

When we love others, as God loves us, we don't simply give what others want. We use our God-given judgment, enlightened by the Holy Spirit, to use our energies and resources to bless others. We lift them up, help them grow and assist them in experiencing the full healing of heart, mind and character to be like Jesus. And often this means that, in love, we say no.

This requires that we exercise our prefrontal cortexes to govern our limbic systems and choose the healthy course of action, despite how it feels. All of life's activities, which strengthen prefrontal-cortex function, prepare us to successfully overcome trying times. Conversely, life experiences that damage the prefrontal cortex and strengthen the limbic system actually set us up for spiritual failure and loss.

In my office, Ellen was breathless with relief. She realized she was right for not wanting to go along with her husband's request. The internal tension was falling, but she wasn't yet free. She wasn't yet ready to successfully deal with her husband because there was one other major distortion operating in her mind—her belief about God's design for marriage.

"But how do I say no, still be obedient to God's Word and submit to my husband like the Bible says?"

"Ellen," I said, "Before we can understand what Paul is dealing with in the New Testament when he gave instructions on wives sub-mitting to their husbands, we must understand God's original design for marriage. Only then can we comprehend what God is trying to accomplish in this world of sin."

I explored with her God's original design for marriage, why God said, "It is not good for the man to be alone. I will make a helper suitable for him" (Gen 2:18). Sadly, throughout history, far too many people have, like Ellen, interpreted this text to mean the woman was made to be Adam's "helper"—just to carry his tools, clean his clothes and cook his meals. But this is wrong. Sin, not God, caused the hor-rible subjugation of women throughout earth's history. The Creator's design was very, very different.

The human race was created in God's image, to love like God loves. It was not good for Adam to be alone, because Adam could not enter into the fullness of Godlike love without someone for Adam to serve, without someone for whom Adam could sacrifice himself, without someone to whom Adam could give himself. Eve was created to be the recipient of Adam's selfless love, and after receiving that love, return it freely in other-centered giving. Adam could never fully live without Eve, to whom he could give himself in loving service. It was God's design, through this powerful, other-centered giving, that two shall become one—one in heart, mind, purpose, devotion and loyalty—one circle of perpetual love.

"Why have I never heard this before?" Ellen asked, a touch of anger in her voice. "Why don't they teach this in church?"

"Because sin is the result of believing lies about God, which break the circle of love and trust," I explained. "Sin broke the bonds of love and infected the hearts and minds of human beings with fear and selfishness. Insecure people want to control others. And we tend to carry out practices in the manner we believe God behaves. If we believe in an authoritarian god, then we usually become controlling toward others."

Ellen nodded as I continued, "It was only after sin that inequality appeared between husband and wife. Any subordination of one partner to the other was not part of God's original design, nor is it part of his healing solution. As we experience more and more of God's healing power in our lives, as selfishness is purged and love is restored within the marriage relationship, we return more fully to God's original ideal—true and genuine equality. *Each* partner sacrifices to uplift the other, to promote the welfare of the other, and to protect the other. Any teaching that perpetuates inequality of moral worth, value, or standing in God's design or service misrepresents God and works against his plan to heal humankind back to his original ideal."

Ellen loved what I was telling her, but she needed scriptural evidence. She needed to see this truth from God's Word, so I handed her my Bible and asked her to read Ephesians 5:21-25:

> Submit to one another out of reverence for Christ. Wives, submit to your own husbands as to the Lord. For the husband is the head of the wife as Christ is the head of the church, his body, of which he is the Savior. Now as the church submits to Christ, so also wives should submit to their husbands in everything. Husbands, love your wives, just as Christ loved the church and gave himself up for her.

"Ellen," I said, "in the first sentence, who is being instructed to submit to whom?"

She reread the words silently, then asked, "Both the husband and wife are to submit to each other?"

"Exactly!" I said. "Then Paul goes on to say that wives are to submit to their husbands, but notice that the husband is to treat his wife like Christ treats the church. How does Christ treat the church?"

Ellen thought for a moment, then looked up at me sharply. "He sacrifices himself," she said.

"Absolutely! The Bible is teaching that wives are *not* to submit blindly to their husbands but are to submit to Christlike treatment from their husbands. Christ led by example, presenting truth in love and leaving people free to think and decide for themselves. Christ gave of himself. He came not to be served but to serve. Therefore, a husband who wants to use this passage to invoke submission from his wife must first be like Jesus. He must put his wife first, build her up, and promote her welfare, happiness and dreams. He must use Christlike methods of presenting truth in love and leave her free, ultimately sacrificing his own happiness, his very life if necessary, to protect the health and happiness of his wife. How does that sound to you?"

"Like a different world." She paused, then added, "You mean I am not supposed to do what he says because he is the husband and I am his wife?"

"What is the greatest of all the commandments?" I asked.

"To love the Lord with all my heart, mind, soul and strength."

"Absolutely. And what is the second greatest commandment?"

"To love my neighbor as myself."

"Does a spouse fall into the God category or your closest neighbor category?"

"My closest neighbor," she said.

I leaned forward in my chair. "Ellen, our first responsibility is always to God. And God has given you your own unique individuality, identity, and ability to think and to reason for yourself. He doesn't want you to surrender your mind to anyone but him—and only to him for healing, not control. He wants to heal your faculties, cleanse your conscience, ennoble your reason and set you free to think for yourself. God expects you to intelligently choose to do what you know is right, healthy and reasonable, because it is right, healthy and reasonable. He doesn't want you to let someone else—even your husband—tell you what to think or do. Jesus even said, 'Those who come to me cannot be my disciples unless they love me more than they love father and mother, wife and children, brothers and sisters, and themselves as well' (Lk 14:26 GNT). We must put God before all others, including our spouse."

As Ellen embraced the truth, her demeanor changed. The tears dried up, the fear and panic subsided, and a dignified calm overcame her. She was composed and somber as she realized what she needed to do. I encouraged her to not just understand the truth, not just comprehend it, but to go home and *apply* this truth to how she interacted with her husband.

When she came back the following week she was completely transformed. She was bright, smiling, bubbling over with joy. She could hardly wait to tell me what happened.

"I told him that I loved him too much to go along with his birthday request. I told him that I couldn't stand by idly and watch as he damaged his mind, character and soul. I told him that I loved him, God and myself too much to go along with such a horrible act. I told him that I loved him and didn't want to lose him, but if he wanted someone else, our marriage was over."

"Good for you! Excellent!" I affirmed.

But Ellen wasn't through with her story. Her voice softened as she said, "I couldn't believe it, but he started to cry. He told me how sorry he was and asked me to forgive him. He told me he loved me and cherished me even more for standing up to him. We prayed together and he asked God to forgive him, and then we prayed for God's blessing on our marriage. Dr. Jennings, I can't believe it."

In my mind I said, *Thank you, Lord!* I was thankful that her husband responded as he did. But even if he hadn't, she had done what was right. The only hope for her personal health and their marital health was truthfully applying the unwavering law of love. There was no possibility of happiness and health if she would have given in to his request. If she did, his limbic system would have been further inflamed, and his prefrontal cortex would have been damaged. She would have experienced guilt and resentment, and love would have been destroyed. There is only one path of health, life and happiness, and it is the path of love. I was thankful that he was receptive to loving truth for it is only as we apply the truth in love that genuine healing occurs.

But love doesn't win everyone. My own heart carries scars of battles lost, divorce, broken friendships, fractured churches. Not all relationships reconcile, even when our love is pure. I thought of God and, despite his perfect love, the many children lost, never to be reconciled. Lost, because what God wants cannot be forced. It can only be freely given.

APPLICATION

If you have ever struggled with fear and insecurity, tempted to act against your conscience in order to win human approval, here are some simple steps that may help:

1. Mentally take a step back and ask, What is the truth? What is the right, healthy and reasonable action for me to take?

2. If someone rejects you or becomes angry with you for doing what you believe is right, ask yourself if that person is really your friend. Do you really want his or her approval?

3. Ask yourself if you are willing to set others free—free to think or feel any way they choose about you. Or are you, on some level, trying to control what others think about you? Are you thinking, *If I do what they want then they won't be mad at me?* Consider setting them free to think whatever they want. And the beauty of God's law of liberty is, when you set others free to think whatever they choose about you, you have just set yourself free from the pressure of conforming to their opinion.

Remember, love does what is right, healthy and reasonable, because it is so, not because it feels good in the moment. So, look beyond the immediate to the principles of God's kingdom, and apply those principles even if it feels uncomfortable in the moment.

Each of these steps involves putting the prefrontal cortex in charge of processing, modulating and, ultimately, ruling over the emotions of the limbic system. God's methods strengthen the prefrontal cortex, improve our ability to think clearly and love fully, whereas allowing the fear circuits to overrule our prefrontal cortex results in an unhealthy and imbalanced brain.

Changing Our View of God

Power is of two kinds. One is obtained by
the fear of punishment and the other by acts of love.
Power based on love is a thousand times more
effective and permanent than the one
derived from fear of punishment.

MAHATMA GANDHI

LAURA CAME TO SEE ME WITH A long history of depression and anxiety. She worried about everything—how people would treat her, whether she would have money to pay her bills, whether she would keep her job, whether her friends really liked her. She had chronic fear of abandonment and intense feelings of loneliness. But she was most terrified of losing people she cared about, so she never let herself get too close. She was married but unhappy. Had children but experienced conflicts. Was employed, but hated her job. Laura had been treated with a variety of medications, all without significant improvement.

She was unhappy with her life, unhappy with her circumstances. There was an undercurrent of anger brewing beneath the surface of her fear and discouragement. When I asked her if she believed in God, she responded with a look of rage mixed with hurt and pain. "Don't you dare talk to me about God," she said, adding that, while she doubted his existence, she was very angry with him. Laura told me that for her entire life she had felt persecuted, punished and beaten up by God. Whenever something bad happened in her life, she would see God doing it to her. She never allowed herself to get her hopes up because she believed that, at any moment, God would step in and ruin her joy. She said she didn't believe in God, yet she hated him and feared him.

As we explored her life history, she told me that when she was seven years old her mother had been killed in an automobile accident. She cried hard as she recounted this painful experience. She told me about her mother and how, after these many years, she still missed her. Then she told me of the funeral, of sitting on the front pew of the church as the preacher looked straight at her and said, "God took your mommy to be with him." Turning toward me with anger burning in her eyes she said, "But I needed my mommy with me!"

Her words echoed in my mind. *But I needed my mommy with me!* What had that well-meaning preacher done? What kind of God was presented to Laura when she was most vulnerable? Innocently, inadvertently, a lie about God was implanted into her mind. That lie simply stated: God takes mommies from their children; God is the source of pain, suffering and death. And what is the neurobiological consequence to believing such a lie about God?

Lies believed break the circle of love and trust. Believing such a frightening view of God, Laura's prefrontal cortex sent signals to the amygdala to fire the alarm, rather than calm it. Anxiety and fear increased, reacting back on the prefrontal cortex, causing further threat-based interpretations of life, resulting in more fear and anxiety. Her mind could not be healed until the lies were removed.

For though we live in the world, we do not wage war as the world does. The weapons we fight with are not the weapons of the world. On the contrary, they have divine power to demolish strongholds. We demolish arguments and every pretension that sets itself up against *the knowledge of God*, and we take captive every thought to make it obedient to Christ. (2 Cor 10:3-5, emphasis mine)

Laura's mind had become a stronghold of fear and doubt. Believing lies about God, she had become filled with bitterness, anger and resentment. Love cannot flow where lies about God are lodged. Without the truth about God, the infection of fear and selfishness has no antidote. Her condition only worsened. She was constantly afraid, incapable of experiencing real joy or peace, seeing exploitation and injury at every turn, unable to genuinely trust others. I knew that in order to get well, in order to find peace, Laura must be freed from her oppressive view of God.

I asked her to tell me about the God in whom she didn't believe. She spent several minutes describing a cruel tyrant, a being who arbitrarily abuses his power to inflict pain and suffering on his creatures, a being who must be appeased, a being who doesn't care that children are abused, one who takes mommies away from their children.

After she finished, I looked directly into her eyes and said, "Good for you; I don't believe in him either!" Shocked at such a reply from a Christian psychiatrist, she looked at me skeptically, so I went on to affirm her for rejecting such a hideous conception of God. I commended her for refusing to surrender her thinking and blindly acquiescing to such abusive authority. She began to soften and, over time, as she was comfortable, we began to explore other possibilities about God and why painful events happen—possibilities that slowly reduced her fear and sense of being persecuted, and opened the way for healing.

Lies about God incite fear and activate the inflammatory cascade, damaging brain and body. In order for our minds to heal, we must realize the truth that the Father is on our side. He is our Friend. He is our Savior! Restoration starts by removing the lies and restoring trust. Fortunately, Laura was willing to ask questions, to seek evidence-based answers, but what if she hadn't been? How can lies be removed if questions are not allowed?

NO QUESTIONS PLEASE

Fran was a timid sixty-year-old woman who had come to see me because of chronic fear and anxiety. She had been a Christian her entire life, was active in her church, taught Sunday school and volunteered on mission trips. She had accepted Jesus as her Savior at fourteen years of age and loved him unceasingly. Yet she had struggled throughout her life with a mysterious insecurity—a deep-seated fear, a dark shadow of anxiety hidden in the recesses of her mind. She never spoke of it because she knew it wasn't supposed to be there if she loved and trusted Jesus as her Savior. But there it was. As a result, she was chronically anxious, afraid and insecure.

She had been treated with a variety of anti-anxiety medications and had seen numerous therapists, counselors and physicians, but she had never found peace. Nothing seemed to work. She was desperate.

Fran grew up in a conservative Christian home where the family schedule revolved around church. She attended a private, Christian school, weekly Sunday school, and had regular family worship times. She was taught the importance of faith and believing God's Word, even if, in her limited human mind, it didn't always make sense. She was taught that when you have "faith" you don't need to ask questions, you simply "believe." But Fran *did* have questions, many of them, but was afraid to ask. She was taught that asking questions, investigating the evidence, reasoning out the issues was a sign that one did not have faith, and without faith one could not be saved. So she buried her uncertainties under the guise of faith—but this only caused more questions.

She was constantly battling with her own thoughts, *What kind of a God doesn't want us to ask questions? Does he have something to*

hide? Is he afraid we won't like what we find out about him? Stop
thinking like that! Jesus died for you, and you should trust him. If you
trusted him you wouldn't ask such stupid questions. You don't have
faith, and without faith, you will go to hell. And so the battle in her
mind raged, and she became increasingly fearful of a God who
would burn little girls in hell for asking questions.

Fran's mind was filled with distortions about God. I knew that her
fear and anxiety could not be cured without her coming to a genuine
knowledge of God. As long as she accepted the idea that asking questions revealed a lack of faith, she suspended the use of her prefrontal
cortex. She could not be healed, saved or restored to God's ideal if
she refused to use her prefrontal cortex, for that's where the human
mind comprehends truth, experiences love and communes with
God. We had to demolish the lies about God that were holding Fran
captive so that his love could heal her heart. We had to get her prefrontal cortex active.

We started in Isaiah 1:11 and read about God berating the people of
Israel, not for such things as idolatry, rebelliousness and disobedience.
Instead we found something incredible. God was rebuking his chosen
people for bringing burnt offerings, observing the appointed feast days,
praying to him, observing the sabbath and going to the temple.

God was actually unhappy with them for doing the very rites he
had instructed them to carry out. Why? Because they were not
thinking or reasoning. They were merely carrying out religious observances from rote and didn't understand the meaning the symbolic
service was to teach. They failed to comprehend the principles of
love their ceremonies acted out, and thus failed to help the poor and
the widow. They "did church," but because they were failing to
think, they brought "meaningless offerings" (Is 1:13). Therefore God
told them explicitly, "Come now, let us reason together . . . though
your sins are like scarlet, they shall be as white as snow; though they
are red as crimson, they shall be like wool" (Is 1:18 NIV 1984).

I pointed at the text and told Fran that a God of love has nothing to hide. He enjoys conversing with his children and eagerly invites our questions. Rituals are the tools he uses to get us to think and to stimulate conversation with him. When the mind is brought into contact with the divine, we come in contact with the source of all truth. When we reason with God, the darkness is expelled, our hearts open in trust, our sinfulness is cleansed, and we are made pure.

As the meaning of that text penetrated Fran's long-held fear, I saw a change come over her. A tiny spark lit inside her, and a flame of hope sprang to life. I could see her mind asking, *Could it really be true?* She wanted more.

I had her read Romans 14:5, "Each of them should be fully convinced in their own mind." And Hebrews 5:14, "But solid food is for the mature, who by constant use have trained themselves to distinguish good from evil." Then I asked her, "How can we be fully convinced in our own minds if we don't think, if we don't ask questions, if we don't examine the evidence? How do we train ourselves to distinguish good from evil if we won't inquire, if we refuse to search for the truth?"

The door to her mind was almost open. The dam holding back a lifetime of pent-up questions was about to burst. It needed only one more nudge. I had her read the words of Jesus himself in John 15:15: "I'm no longer calling you servants because servants *don't under-stand* what their master is thinking and planning. No, I've named you friends because I've let you in on everything I've heard from the Father" (*The Message*, emphasis mine).

Fran saw it: Jesus doesn't want us to be unthinking servants who just do what we are told. He wants us to be his intelligent, under-standing friends who think for ourselves, who have recovered the ability to discern right from wrong. The floodgate burst open. Questions began to pour out.

But one question plagued Fran more than any other. It's a question that has troubled many of my other patients as well, an idea that undermines trust in God. It had to be resolved before she could find peace.

"GOD DON'T MAKE NO JUNK"

"Why did God make me this way?" Fran asked. "Why did God want me to have anxiety and depression?" She told me she believed God uses his divine power to create each of us as individuals, just as we are. She even had a shirt once that said, "God made me, and God don't make no junk!"

Here was another very subtle distortion that had crept into her thinking. It was causing mental distress and undermining trust in God. She believed the lie that God directly creates each one of us just as we are, complete with all of our genetic flaws, diseases, defects and sin. However, the Bible does not teach this idea. It teaches that the human species was created by God perfect and sinless.

When God created Adam and Eve in the Garden of Eden, he not only made them flawless, he also gave them the ability to pro-create (Gen 1:28). God created them with freedom to choose and change or adapt based on their choices. This means the very choices of Adam and Eve would change them. Healthy choices would result in greater development and health, but deviations from the law of love would result in defect, damage and, without intervention, eventual death. Once they turned their backs on God and sinned, all of their offspring have been "sinful at birth, sinful from the time my mother conceived me" (Ps 51:5). In other words, all humanity has been born defective.

Many of my patients have struggled in their relationships with God because they have believed the lie that God created them, as individuals, exactly as they are. They ask, "Why did God want me to be schizophrenic?" "Why did God want my child to have autism?" "Why did God create me with bipolar disorder?"

Truth is, he didn't! God doesn't use his power to create sinful, sick, defective and deformed beings. All defects are a result of sin contaminating and damaging God's creation. Love does not—cannot—create imperfection.

Fran was not initially convinced on this point, so she asked more questions. "But what about where the Bible says, 'For you created my inmost being; you knit me together in my mother's womb'?" (Ps 139:13).

"Excellent!" I responded. "Good for you. Don't accept someone else's ideas. Think for yourself. Ask questions and reason out the issues. You have cited a Bible passage. But quoting a verse is not enough. We must ask, 'What does it mean?'"

She was not used to this. She had been taught, "If the Bible says it, I believe it and that settles it." She realized, however, that such an approach shut down thinking, prevented reasoning, and impaired her ability to actually know God and appreciate how he works. So she began to think, *What does it mean?* This activated her prefrontal cortex and opened her mind to the Holy Spirit.

I had already explained God's law of love and the ongoing battle with the satanic infection. We had explored how all nature was suffering under the weight of sin, but these were new concepts she struggled to incorporate into her thinking.

I continued, "If God is the one who is directly creating each individual human being, then when children are born with congenital heart defects, spina bifida, deformities of various kinds, is God having a bad 'knitting' day? Are we comfortable laying at God's feet all genetic defects and deformities? If God is directly creating babies with congenital defects, then when doctors do surgery to save the lives of infants, are they opposing the divine will? Should health care professionals refuse to repair birth defects, claiming God wants certain people born that way? If God is the one using his power to create each of us, then is his power weaker than a sinful human mother who drinks so much alcohol that her baby is born with fetal alcohol syndrome? If God is actively creating that baby, shouldn't his power be greater than the alcohol being consumed by the thoughtless mother, and shouldn't the child be born healthy in spite of it?"

Fran looked to be struggling with these new ideas, but I pressed on. "Worse yet, if we believe that God is directly creating each individual human, then during the anarchy in Sudan when Arab men went around raping Sudanese women by the tens of thousands in order to have more children of Arab descent, should those women turn to God and thank him for what just happened? Is rape how God creates? Does the law of love include rape?

"More serious than physical deformity and rape, do we believe God actually creates sin and sinners? If we say that God creates us as individuals by his direct power, and we realize that each of us is born sinful, then we are saying that God creates sinners."

Fran knew this could not be true. She realized that the Bible gives God credit for directly creating only two human lives—Adam and Eve—and later Jesus' incarnation. All three of them were sinless. Jesus remained that way. Adam and Eve did not.

Fran's mind was processing, working to integrate truth and weed out distortion. She looked over at me and asked, "Then how do we understand God's role in our individual creation?"

I was ready with my answer. "When God gave Samson strength, did God control how Samson used that strength? When God gave Solomon wisdom, did God control how Solomon used that gift? When God gave the human species the ability to procreate, does God decide where and with whom we mate? Does God control the use of his gifts, or does God give us abilities, talents and opportunities, and then leave us free to use them for good or evil as we so choose?"

Fran had never considered these possibilities before, and this was hard work for someone used to believing without thinking. So I continued slowly and prayerfully. "God is the one who gave Samson strength, but God is not the one who chose to use that strength to philander with heathen women. God is the one who gave Solomon wisdom, but God is not the one who chose to use that wisdom to marry seven hundred wives or make altars to idols. God has given the human race the ability to create, but he does not control how we use that ability.

"God is the Creator of the design template of humanity as well as the laws of nature and physics that govern reproduction. So he is the one 'knitting together' through his ordained design and laws. But he is not directly creating each of us with sin, disease and defect." I reminded my patient that our current condition is a result of God's creation being infected with sin, that all nature groans under the weight of sin (Rom 8:22).[1]

When Fran finally saw the truth—that love was battling with selfishness, that God did not create her with sin, disease and defects, but has been working to save and heal her—her fear and distrust of him began to vanish. Incredible new possibilities began to open before her mind. The fresh air of freedom finally blew into her soul—freedom to think, freedom to ask questions, freedom to choose. And as freedom swept in and her love and appreciation for God grew, fear faded away.

The Bible exploded with new meaning for Fran. When she read about the woman caught in adultery and heard Jesus say, "Neither do I condemn you," she heard the voice of the Father. When she read of Jesus washing the feet of his betrayer, she saw the Father bending over sinners to wash away sin. When she saw Jesus allowing an angry mob to beat him, spit on him and crucify him, she saw the face of God receiving the blows, dripping with blood, dying in agony When she read Jesus' invitation to be his friend (Jn 15:15) she felt the love of the Father calling her home.

Many of us have been lied to about God. When we believe those lies, the circle of love and trust becomes broken in our hearts, and fear and selfishness quickly take hold. The more deeply rooted the lies, the greater the fear. But the story doesn't have to end there. The way to restored love is always through the path of rediscovered truth.

9

The Power of Truth

Truth indeed rather alleviates than hurts,
and will always bear up against falsehood,
as oil does above water.

MIGUEL DE CERVANTES

JOE WAS DYING OF COLON CANCER. It was too late for treatment; the cancer was too far spread to heal. Joe told me he noticed some rectal bleeding four years earlier, but rather than going to the doctor to get an evaluation, he told himself, "It must be hemorrhoids." He was afraid of the possibility of what rectal bleeding could mean. The thought of having cancer was too emotionally distressing, so rather than pursuing the truth, he attempted to avoid it. But as Joe learned all too well, we can never avoid the truth—we can only delay the day we'll have to deal with it. Delaying pursuit of the truth does not prevent the truth from happening. Delay only makes the problem worse when we are finally forced to face it.

Sadly, far too many people fail to realize that the ultimate reason for pursuing the truth: healing. Instead, throngs of people fear the truth. They fear that knowing the truth will cause pain, embarrassment or loss—of position, job, respect, health, relationship or reputation. So they run from it. But we must learn to be truthful in all things, in all circumstances, in all relationships, for truth destroys lies and opens the life for healing.

If we deal with the truth right now, here on this earth, we will still experience life's storms, but we'll deal with them under the comforting umbrella of God's grace, with all the agencies of heaven on our side, working to heal and restore us to mental, emotional and spiritual wellness. But if we deny the truth, run from it, suppress it or even ignore it, we only delay the moment in which we'll have to deal with it. If we delay long enough, we will pass the point of recovery, whether physical or spiritual.

SINCERITY IS NOT SUFFICIENT

Greg was a twenty-three-year-old man who was admitted to the intensive care unit with a blood sugar over one thousand. He was in a condition called diabetic ketoacidosis—a life-threatening condition caused by not taking his insulin. Greg had been a diabetic since childhood. He had been hospitalized many times in the past and knew the dangers of stopping his insulin. Therefore, after he was medically stabilized, a psychiatric consult was obtained to determine if he was suicidal, if he was purposely refusing his treatment in an attempt to kill himself.

Greg told me he had no desire to die but had stopped his insulin because he had been "healed." He enthusiastically described a "revival" he had recently attended at a local church. During the event, those with sickness and illness were invited to come forward. Loud and emotional prayers were made, hands were laid on him, and an invocation for healing was delivered: "In the name of the Lord Jesus Christ, be healed!" His emotions soared with exhilaration and he sincerely believed he'd been healed. He had never "felt" so good, he told me, so he stopped taking his insulin. Now he was in the ICU at death's door. The truth of his condition was contradicting his sincerely held belief. Sincerity—convincing oneself that something is true despite the evidence—is not the same as resting on truth. Those who value truth, know miracles can, and do, happen. But because they love truth, they are not afraid to examine the evidence that demonstrates that healing has actually occurred (Heb 5:14). Bottom line, no matter how we "feel," if we reject the truth we cannot get well.

Brain imaging studies have demonstrated that religious practices such as Greg experienced inflame limbic-system structures and reduce activity in the prefrontal cortex. Since truth enters our minds via the neural circuits of the prefrontal cortex, it is not surprising that the powerful emotional experiences by Greg resulted in his inability to make a reasonable, truth-based decision. The Holy Spirit is the Spirit of truth and always works in harmony with, never against, the truth. When the Holy Spirit is involved, the prefrontal cortex becomes healthier, the ability to reason improves, and love, compassion and empathy grow stronger. When false "spirits"—sometimes identified as feelings—are involved, prefrontal-cortex activity is impaired, the limbic system is inflamed, and reason, love and compassion are undermined. We cannot be healed until we accept the truth.[1]

WE MUST APPLY THE TRUTH

Jesse was in the ICU, heavily sedated, on a ventilator and could not communicate in any way. He was fifty-nine, but he looked eighty. He was dirty, unshaven and unwashed with nicotine-stained fingers. A foul cocktail of body odors mixed with tobacco hung in the air. Jesse was severely malnourished. His skin hung loosely from his bones; his eyes were sunk deep into the sockets, and the whites of his eyes were a dark, eerie yellow with blood dots speckled throughout. If it wasn't for the ventilator causing his chest to rise and fall and the monitor showing a constant heart rhythm, he could easily be mistaken for dead. But he wasn't dead—not yet, anyway.

As I was unable to get any history from Jesse, I reviewed his chart. It revealed that he was in liver failure, had severe electrolyte problems, resulting in a recent seizure, complete with cardiac arrhythmias, and he was bleeding from his gastrointestinal system. All of this damage had been caused by years of heavy alcohol use. Jesse's life was literally hanging in the balance.

The attending physician had told me, "This guy is an alcoholic, and if we are able to save him, he's going to need rehab."

Seven days later Jesse was off the ventilator, his electrolytes had been stabilized, the bleeding stopped, his liver was working again—just barely—and the detoxification from alcohol was progressing well enough that his mind was now clearer so that he could engage in meaningful conversation. I entered his room and extended my hand. "Hello, I'm Dr. Jennings. I'm a psychiatrist and your doctor has asked me to see you."

"I don't need no psychiatrist!" Jesse responded with disdain.

"Do you know where you are?" I asked.

"In the hospital. I ain't crazy."

"No one said you were. I just want to check your memory and see if any of these medicines are affecting your thinking. Do you know why you're here?"

"I been drinking."

"How much?"

"Nuff to get drunk."

"And how much is that?"

"A fifth."

"A fifth of what?"

He offered no evasive answer and shot back, "Whisky, Jim Beam whisky. Sure use some right now."

"Why do you think you could use some whisky right now?"

"So I can get drunk."

"Do you think your drinking has anything to do with why you're here?"

"Of course it do. I 'spect I'll die from drinkin'. Gotta die from som'ing."

I looked at my patient for a long moment. "Your doctor wants me to evaluate you for admission to an alcohol rehab program once you're stable enough to leave the ICU. It's a place that will help you learn how to stay sober so you won't die from drinking. Have you ever been in a rehab program before?"

"I ain't going to no rehab program!" he said angrily.

"Have you ever been to a rehab program before?"

"Four or five. Can't 'member. But I ain't going to no rehab!"

"If you don't go to rehab, where are you going to go?"

"Home."

"Who do you live with?"

"Myself."

"You live alone?"

"You heard me."

"What are your plans when you leave here?"

"Same as they were before I came. I'm gonna get drunk."

"Do you want to die? Are you trying to kill yourself?"

"No, I don't want to die, and I ain't trying to kill myself neither!" he said, annoyed.

"What do you think will happen if you go home and drink?"

"It'll 'ventually kill me I 'spect."

Somewhat confused and searching for clarity, I pressed on. "If you don't want to die and you know drinking is going to kill you, then why are you planning to go home and drink?"

"Cause I like gettin' drunk. I like how it feels. I like it more than most anything in life I 'spect, and I'd rather die than not drink."

Dazed with disbelief at what I was hearing, I remembered something I'd learned earlier in my career: *Insight does not equal change.* Knowing the truth is not sufficient, we must not only know it, we must apply it to our lives if we want healing, if we want to get well. Jesse understood all too clearly that alcohol was killing him, that he needed to stop if he wanted to live, but he was unwilling to apply this truth to his life. In fact, he actively refused to apply the truth and instead chose the path of willful self-destruction.

I saw it so clearly. Jesse's situation was a microcosm of our sin-sick state. At that moment, my heart empathized with God. How he must hurt! Here were all these doctors, nurses, respiratory therapists, social workers, physical therapists and nutritionists working to save, heal and remedy this poor man. There was no condemnation. None of the health-care team was seeking to punish. No one needed appeasement in order to minister to Jesse. All the resources the hospital and medical community could provide were being poured out to redeem this gentleman, and it was heartbreaking to realize there was ultimately nothing we could do to save him. Jesse was so settled into his self-destructive way that, while he would accept interventions to relieve immediate suffering, while he would drain hundreds of thousands of dollars of resources to keep himself well enough to drink, he refused all treatments that would actually transform his life and cure him.

God has poured out all the agencies of heaven for our healing. He has sent angels, seraphim and cherubim, legions of heavenly host, and his Spirit to guide, comfort and heal. Then, in an act of astonishing selflessness, he sent his Son to win the victory we could not. God is not seeking to punish. He is not condemning and doesn't need appeasement to heal and save. All of heaven is emptied for our rescue, for our restoration. Yet, like Jesse, far too many of God's children are so settled into their self-destructive habits that they refuse his remedy.

When in pain, when times are tough, when sin's destructive weight eventually comes crushing down, many turn to God for *momentary* relief or escape from the pain, but then refuse to follow God's prescriptions that would actually transform and cure them for eternity. Just like Jesse and his Jim Beam, far too many seek God's power, resources and grace, not for salvation or genuine healing, but merely to provide the means to continue living their self-destructive lives. How heartbroken God must be realizing that, for some, because of their refusal, there is ultimately nothing he can do to save them.

10

The Truth About Sin

All truths are easy to
understand once they are discovered;
the point is to discover them.

GALILEO

SAVANNAH, THE FIFTEEN-YEAR-OLD PATIENT discussed in chapter 6, came to her following appointment still struggling with fear, continuing to worry about God, and feeling too sinful to be accepted. She wouldn't be able to find total peace until greater truth was understood. The avenue of love was obstructed by misunderstanding, so I continued my questions. "What is sin?" I asked after she'd settled comfortably into her chair.

"Doing bad stuff," she responded.

"How do you know what bad stuff is?"

She had been educated in private, Christian schools her entire life and was confident she knew this answer. "By the Ten Commandments."

"And what makes sin wrong?"

"God said not to do it."

"Why did God say not to do it?"

"Because it's . . . wrong?"

I could see we were starting to circle, so I asked, "And what if you disobey God and do what he says not to do?"

"He has to punish you."

"Do you believe God has to punish you for what you have done?"

She looked confused, "I hope not." Then added, "But if I don't accept the blood of Jesus for my sins he will."

"What would God do to you if Jesus wasn't there offering his blood?"

"He would have to kill me."

"Why?"

"Because in order to be just, God has to punish sin." She had been a good student in her Bible classes and learned these conventional lessons well.

"And what keeps God from punishing sin in your life?"

"Jesus took my place and was punished for me, so if I accept Jesus as my Savior, God doesn't have to punish me." Wow! She really had paid attention. I don't think she would have thought that up on her own.

Leaning forward in my chair I asked, "Savannah, does a God like that scare you?" Without saying a word, she slowly moved her head up and down as a look of apprehension spread across her face. Lies believed break the circle of love and trust, inciting fear and self-ishness. I understood that worshiping an authoritarian, punishing god inflames the fear center (amygdala), damages the prefrontal cortex, and impairs healing and growth. My young patient could never experience wellness as long as lies about God were retained. I knew exactly how she felt. I remember those sleepless nights, those restless days, those years of living afraid of a god who had to be paid in order to be merciful. I knew firsthand she would never really find peace until trust in God was restored.

"Imagine you were born with cystic fibrosis, an inherited and terminal lung disease," I said, "and sometime after birth you developed a cough, fever and chills. So you go to the doctor and, instead of diagnosing cystic fibrosis and lung infection, he diagnoses cough, fever and chills. Would cough, fever and chills be the disease or the symptoms of the disease?"

"Symptoms," she said.

"But what if the doctor treated you with Tylenol for the fever, a cough suppressant for the cough, and warm blankets for the chills . . . and nothing more. Would you get well?"

"No."

"Why not?"

"Because the disease is not being treated; just the symptoms."

"Beautiful!" I said, "In order to get well we have to correctly diagnose the problem and then treat the underlying illness, not just the symptoms, right?"

"Right," she agreed.

I wanted to help her see she didn't need to be afraid of God. So I said, "Jesus taught that the acts of sin—the bad things we do—are not the primary problem, they are the *symptoms* of the problem. In Matthew 5 he says, 'You say when you commit adultery [that's a bad act] you commit sin. I say when you look at another with lust in your heart you have already committed adultery. You say when you commit murder [another bad act] you commit sin. I say when you hate your brother in your heart. . . .' Jesus is teaching that bad acts result from a sin-sick heart, that the bad acts are symptoms, like fever and cough, letting us know that we are spiritually sick and in need of God's healing. Our true diagnosis is our sinful heart, which results in bad acts.

"Is it possible," I continued, "that in Christianity we have misdiagnosed the problem? Is it possible we have believed our problem is our 'sins'—the 'bad acts'—rather than the fearful and selfish heart that leads to bad acts? Is it possible we have misunderstood and failed to realize that our bad behavior is a symptom of a bad heart? And is it possible, having misdiagnosed the problem, that we have created a system designed to treat the symptoms rather than accepting God's remedy to heal the true, underlying illness?"

Savannah looked confused, "I don't understand."

"Have you been afraid God has to punish you for having sex?"

She nodded yes.

"Would you be afraid that your doctor would have to punish you for having fever and cough?"

"No, but I couldn't help it if I was born with cystic fibrosis and had fever and cough. I have a choice when it comes to sin."

"Not without Jesus. Not without the indwelling of the Holy Spirit. In our own human strength we don't have a choice. We are born into sin (Ps 51:5). Just like being born with cystic fibrosis, we are born with a terminal condition that, if not cured, will result in death."

I paused then asked, "Why did you have sex with that young man?"

"Because I was afraid. I didn't want him to be mad at me."

"And when did you choose to have fear and insecurity?"

"I didn't choose it. I've had insecurity my whole life."

"Are you saying that you have a condition of heart—fear and insecurity—you didn't choose, but this insecurity impacts the decisions you make?"

She nodded slowly, her mind processing my words.

"As soon as Adam and Eve sinned, they ran and hid because they were *afraid*. Fear is part of the infection of sin. Every human born since our first parents sinned is born infected with fear and selfishness—a terminal condition—just like being born with cystic fibrosis. We didn't choose to be this way. It isn't our fault, just like being born with cystic fibrosis wouldn't be our fault. But if we don't accept God's remedy, even though it isn't our fault we were born this way, we will still die."

She nodded as she began tracking what I was saying.

"While it wouldn't be your fault if you were born with cystic fibrosis, if there was a free remedy that would cure you and you refused it, would that be your fault?"

"Yes," she said instantly.

"That is the question you need to focus on. Have you accepted God's free remedy that will cure you? The acts of sin, the disobedience we tend to focus on (like having sex outside of marriage) are actually the symptoms of the condition of sinfulness. And like fever and cough, which tell us that something is wrong and that we need medical treatment, our acts of sin reveal our hearts are sick and in need of God's spiritual treatment. Acts of sin are like symptoms from any disease: the longer the disease goes untreated and the more symptoms we have, the more damage we incur and the sicker we get. Therefore, we don't want to minimize the symptoms (our sins) or pretend they are inconsequential, because they're not. The acts of sin damage our minds, sear our consciences, warp our reason, mar our characters, and make it easier and easier to resist God, ultimately resulting in our eternal loss."

I explained the relationship between acts of sin, which strengthen limbic-system circuits and damage prefrontal-cortex circuits, and the increase in fear, guilt and shame. Her eyes were riveted to me as she listened intently.

"Therefore we want to avoid the acts of sin. Yet, like focusing on treating the cough and fever, instead of the underlying illness, when we focus on getting our misdeeds pardoned, our sins appeased, the penalty for our transgressions paid, the record of our sins erased, rather than getting our hearts and minds healed, we actually get worse rather than better. Savannah, God wants so much more than to merely forgive your sins. God wants to completely transform your heart and renew your mind."

I paused to let her think. I knew if she was going to experience God's healing power in her life, we needed to correct many of the ideas she had been taught that made her think God was mad at her, that God was someone she should try to avoid. Love cannot flow where lies about God abound.

"Imagine being sick," I said, trying a slightly different approach, "and going to the doctor. When he comes in to examine you, would you push your healthy brother in front of you and ask the doctor to examine him instead?"

"That wouldn't make any sense," she said with a chuckle.

"Then why do many Christians teach that, for the saved, God doesn't look at them, he looks at Jesus who stands in their place? Yet David prayed, 'Search *me*, God, and know *my* heart; test *me* and know *my* anxious thoughts. See if there is any offensive way in *me*, and lead *me* in the way everlasting.' And 'Create in *me* a pure heart, O God, and renew a steadfast spirit within *me*' (Ps 139:23-24; 51:10, emphasis mine). Shouldn't we want God, just like our doctor, to search us thoroughly, finding every defect of heart, mind and character, and then heal us?"

She nodded.

"You don't need to be afraid of your doctor, and you don't need to be afraid of God. Because God, just like your doctor, just wants to heal you. If you were sick and in the hospital, would you try to get the nurses to erase the medical records so the doctor wouldn't know how sick you were?"

"No," she said.

"Why do we teach that Jesus is erasing the sins of the righteous from the records of heaven?"

"Because we don't want God to see them," she said.

"And why don't we want God to see the record of our sins or to see us the way we are?"

"Because we're afraid of him, because we believe he has to punish us."

She was struggling with deeply indoctrinated ideas so I pressed even harder. "If the doctor came to examine you, would you be afraid to let him?"

"No. I would want him to."

"And if he offered you a treatment that would actually cure you, but you refused to take it, would you be afraid that the doctor, in order to be just, would kill you?"

"No," she said, paused and then, with some excitement in her voice, blurted out, "If I refused the treatment, the *disease* would kill me—not the *doctor!*" She had made an important breakthrough.

I smiled broadly as I reached for my Bible. "And that is exactly how it is with sin. Notice what the Bible says, 'Evil will slay the wicked'; 'The wages of sin is death, but the gift of God is eternal life'; 'Sin, when it is full-grown, gives birth to death'; and 'The one who sows to please his sinful nature, *from that nature* will reap destruction' [Ps 34:21; Rom 6:23; Jas 1:15; Gal 6:8 NIV 1984, emphasis mine]. The Bible teaches that sin, just like cystic fibrosis, if unremedied, results in death. God hates sin like a doctor hates disease because sin destroys those he loves. And God, just like a doctor, loves his sick patients (all of us earth-bound sinners) and is working tirelessly to heal and save.

"The difference between God and your doctor is that your doctor doesn't have someone telling you that he is mean, angry, unforgiving, severe and out to hurt you. God, on the other hand, has an enemy, the father of lies, who is constantly working to misrepresent him, to get us to believe perversity about God so that we won't trust him and, therefore, won't open our hearts to him for genuine healing. Our thinking has become so backward that we are actually more afraid of our spiritual doctor (God) than the sickness (sin) that is killing us!

"Savannah, when you see the truth about God and open your heart in trust to him, he will heal you. He will remove your guilt, restore your dignity, and renew your heart to be like his."

"That's what I want!" she said, her voice echoing the longing in her heart. "I want peace. But how? I don't know how. I don't even know how to pray."

"Prayer is simply talking with God like talking with one of your friends. It is opening your heart to God and telling him *exactly* what you're thinking, feeling, desiring. Prayer is sharing with God the inmost secrets of your life: your dreams, fears, joys and sorrows. Brain research shows that fifteen minutes a day in meditation or thoughtful communion with the God of love results in measurable development of the prefrontal cortex, especially in the anterior cingulate cortex (ACC). This is the area where we experience love, compassion and empathy. The healthier the ACC, the calmer the amygdala (alarm center), and the less fear and anxiety we experience. Truly, love casts out all fear! If you want God to heal you, if you want his presence, forgiveness and grace, all you have to do is tell him, give him permission to come into your heart, and then spend thoughtful time in communion with him each and every day."

Savannah isn't the only one struggling with guilt, fear and insecurity, searching for peace. Since Adam and Eve's fall, all humanity has been struggling. But if the diagnosis is wrong, the treatment is usually wrong. Healing starts when we finally acknowledge our sin condition, realize the truth about God and surrender ourselves to him. Until then, the symptoms only worsen.

Enlarging Our View of God

A PASTOR FRIEND OF MINE grew up on a farm in the Upper Peninsula of Michigan in the 1950s. It was a quiet, rural area with great distances between family farms, but the neighbors were friendly and everyone knew each other by name. His closest neighbors had several children. The youngest, Bobby, was age five when the following events transpired.

It was common for boys who grew up on farms to start working at a very young age. It would not be unusual to see a young man of twelve driving a tractor, plowing the fields or delivering feed to the cattle. But generally children of age five were not allowed around the farm equipment.

From an early age Bobby was difficult. As an infant he was inconsolable, as a toddler he would frequently throw tantrums, and as a child he was out of control. When told to pick up his toys, he would do so with back talk or not at all. He was frequently caught stealing cookies or candy, and he often took toys that were not his. He was instructed repeatedly by his parents to never, ever play around the farm equipment. They even threatened him with spanking if they ever caught him near the dangerous machinery, which they had to enforce on more than one occasion. But Bobby was an unruly, disobedient child.

One day when my friend was fifteen years old, he received word while working in the fields that Bobby had been injured. The neighbors were asking that his family come and pray for him. Bobby had been playing around the farm equipment and sustained serious, life-threatening injuries. In the 1950s in the Upper Peninsula of Michigan there was no 911 to call, no Life Force helicopter to swoop down from the sky, no emergency responders waiting close by, so the family did the only thing they knew how to do. They called their neighbors, formed a prayer circle around Bobby and asked for God's intervention.

My friend told me of his vivid memory of that day. One by one, neighbor after neighbor prayed for Bobby, a prayer that went something like this: "Lord, Bobby is hurt. His life is hanging in the balance. We know you can heal, you can restore, you can save his life. We come to you humbly now and ask, if it be your will, please restore Bobby to health." Prayer after prayer ended just like that: "If it be your will, your will be done . . ."

Then it was time for Bobby's mother to pray. She said simply, "God, I don't care what your will is. If you don't heal my son, I will never speak to you again."

What happened after that is a matter of history, so I will report it to you. Bobby survived and grew up to be a blight on that family and community. He was constantly in trouble, disobedient to his parents and rebellious at school. He got into vandalism, truancy, petty theft, alcohol and drugs. He stole money and property from his parents and neighbors and pawned it for drugs, and was in and out of jail his entire life.

We are not currently privileged to see with perfect, eternal vision. We don't know whether God intervened to save Bobby or whether Bobby recovered on his own. But this story gives us opportunity to ask questions, to explore possibilities, to consider life from a larger view.

Why was Bobby, at age five, in a life-threatening situation? Did God act to threaten Bobby's life, or were his injuries a direct consequence of his own actions? Is it possible that God intervened to save Bobby's life? Is it possible God knew the heart of that mother and understood that she would close her heart to him if he didn't save Bobby, and since God didn't want to lose her, he intervened? Is it possible that, if the mother would have trusted God and prayed, "God, I don't want to lose my son, but I don't know the future. I don't know how life will unfold; I don't know what is best. But I do know you always do what is best. So, Father, I trust you. Please heal my son if it is in your will," that Bobby might not have survived? Is it possible his survival was from a lack of trust in God, not from a great trust in God? If the mother had trusted God, is it possible that the Almighty, knowing the future, might not have intervened to save Bobby and instead allowed him to die from the natural consequence of his injuries, thus sparing years of heartache to so many people, including Bobby himself?

We don't know whether or not God intervened to save Bobby, but this story gives us opportunity to step back and enlarge our perspective when dealing with pain, trauma and loss in our lives.

MIRACLES AND FAITH

Harold was a quiet, thirty-seven-year-old man referred for evaluation by his oncologist for possible depression related to end-of-life issues. Even though he was a young man, Harold was dying. He had been diagnosed with an aggressive esophageal cancer several months before and was undergoing treatment, but his prognosis was poor.

Harold was happily married and had three beautiful children, ages ten, seven and five. Understandably, he didn't want to die and was quite tempted with powerful feelings: feelings of fear, deep sadness and despair. The diagnosis of cancer inflamed his amygdala, resulting in his prefrontal cortex ruminating on fear-inducing themes. But Harold didn't want to surrender to despair, he didn't want to be controlled by his feelings, and he certainly didn't want to get sucked into the pit of depression. If these were to be his last days on earth, he wanted to live them as fully and productively as possible. That's why he came to see me.

Although Harold was a Christian and presented himself with a courageous perspective, he still had doubts, still struggled with fears and still battled with uncertainty. *How could this happen to me? What did I do to deserve this? I have been a Christian my entire life. I haven't committed any really bad sins. Why me? God knows my children need me. Why should I have to die?*

Harold was struggling to internalize and deal effectively with the truth. He had gone to a healing ceremony at his church, a ceremony where he was anointed with oil while the pastor and elders laid hands on him and asked for God's miraculous intervention. That was two weeks prior to our appointment. But Harold was no better. At his follow-up medical visits, the doctors found no improvement; in fact, the cancer was continuing to progress. This caused more doubt, more fear and more uncertainty.

Why didn't God heal me? I know he can. He has healed others. Why not me? Am I not saved? Am I not good enough? Do I lack faith? Is there some unknown sin in my life? Am I being punished? Why wasn't I healed?

Harold would never find the truth to heal his mind until he enlarged his perspective. I started by sharing with him an experience I had some years before.

During my freshman year at a Christian college a rather unusual event occurred one Thursday morning when, during chapel, the entire student body came face-to-face with the question of faith and miracles. A young man who was a quadriplegic from a diving accident was brought into the chapel. The speaker instructed the students that we were going to see a miracle—God was going to heal this young man. He told all two thousand of us to kneel and pray. He told us to prayerfully clear our hearts of any sin, remove any doubt from our minds and any distraction from our consciousness. Then he told us to pray that God would miraculously heal this young man.

Harold was listening intently to my story, so I continued.

The preacher and several others gathered around the paralyzed man and placed hands on him and then began to pray. We students prayed and prayed and prayed. There were girls crying all over the auditorium. Some students were praying out loud, others were sneaking peaks at the stage, watching to see a "miracle." After what seemed like hours, but in fact was twenty-five minutes, no miracle happened and the young man was not healed.

Looking at Harold I said, "Many of the students were shaken by this event. Some struggled with questions about their faith, about prayer and about God himself. The speaker suggested there were doubters in the room, and some students began to feel guilty. Have you struggled with questions about God and faith since your cancer was discovered, since you have not been healed?"

"Yes," he said, "I've had all those questions."

"There is an unstated belief within many Christian groups," I said: "If you have faith, miracles will happen, and if miracles don't happen, it is because faith is weak. But is this really true? Is the idea that miracles happen when faith is strong, but not when weak, a biblical one? Or is it possible that this idea could be almost 180 degrees backward from the truth? Is it possible that miracles happen not for the strong in faith but for the weak? Is it possible that those whose faith is solid don't need the miracles, but the 'babes' in Christ still need miraculous signs and wonders? Is it possible that miracles often occur *through* the strong in faith but not *for* the strong in faith, that the purpose of the miracle is for those weak in faith?"

Harold wasn't sure. He liked the general direction of my questions but needed some evidence to help him see the wider view more clearly.

"What does the Bible reveal?" I asked. "When Gideon was called by God to defeat the Midianites, did he ask for the miracles of the fleece because his faith was strong or because his faith was weak and he needed encouragement?"

"He needed encouragement," Harold agreed.

"At Mount Carmel, fire fell from God, consuming the sacrifice offered by Elijah. Was this great miracle given for Elijah to strengthen his faith, or was the miracle given for the people who were weak in faith?"

"The miracle was for the people who were weak in faith." Harold saw the lesson quite clearly.

Then I brought up Job, who God said was "blameless and upright," with "no one on earth like him" (Job 1:8). Job was a real man of faith, yet he lost all his wealth, his health and ten children. No miracle delivered him. Did this tragedy happen to Job because his faith was weak, I asked, or did it occur because his faith was so strong that God knew nothing, no matter how tragic, could shake Job out of trusting him?

I went on with another example. "When Shadrach, Meshach and Abednego were thrown into the fiery furnace, God miraculously intervened to save their lives, but for what purpose? Was it primarily to extend the lives of the men thrown into the furnace, or was it a means of exposing the impotence of the golden idol, showing the truth about God and reaching Nebuchadnezzar, a man weak in faith? By contrast, notice the genuine, mature faith of the three worthies who, when threatened with a burning death, put their lives into God's hands and trusted him with the outcome, knowing God could save but allowing God not to intervene. They said, 'King Nebuchadnezzar, we do not need to defend ourselves before you in this matter. If we are thrown into the blazing furnace, the God we serve is able to deliver us from it, and he will deliver us from Your Majesty's hand. *But even if he does not*, we want you to know, Your Majesty, that we will not serve your gods or worship the image of gold you have set up'" (Dan 3:16-18, emphasis mine).

Harold was thinking. The wheels were turning. His prefrontal cortex was working, so I continued. "Consider the lives of the apostles. God miraculously intervened in many places but always as a means of spreading the gospel. God did not miraculously intervene to save these mighty men of faith—with the exception of John. Did God refuse to perform miracles to save his apostles because they didn't have enough faith, or was their faith so strong that they trusted God with their very lives? Was their faith so intense that God didn't have to perform a miracle to help them maintain their confidence in him?"

Harold nodded, "Yes, I can see their faith in God was so strong that they didn't need a miracle to keep them faithful, but why didn't God just deliver them because he loved them? I would save my child from illness if I could. Why doesn't God?"

"Excellent question," I affirmed. "Let's reexamine the story of Job, which gives some insight into that question. Where does the setting in the book of Job begin?"

"In heaven," Harold said.

"Exactly, after telling us a little bit about Job—where he is from, how many children he has and so on—the Bible shifts the view to heaven." I read a few verses to Harold:

> One day the angels came to present themselves before the LORD, and Satan also came with them. The LORD said to Satan, "Where have you come from?"
>
> Satan answered the LORD, "From roaming throughout the earth, going back and forth on it."
>
> Then the LORD said to Satan, "Have you considered my servant Job? There is no one on earth like him; he is blameless and upright, a man who fears God and shuns evil."

"Does Job fear God for nothing?" Satan replied. "Have you not put a hedge around him and his household and everything he has? You have blessed the work of his hands, so that his flocks and herds are spread throughout the land. But now stretch out your hand and strike everything he has, and he will surely curse you to your face."

The LORD said to Satan, "Very well, then, everything he has is in your power, but on the man himself do not lay a finger."

Then Satan went out from the presence of the LORD. (Job 1:6-12)

After reading, I asked Harold what was happening in the scene.

"God is having a gathering of his intelligent creatures from around the universe, and Satan shows up from planet Earth."

"Right," I said. "And did you notice what God did? He made a judgment. He judged Job to be upright, or righteous, and some translations say 'perfect in all his ways.' And then Satan says, 'Wait just one minute. He only pretends to be good, pretends to be righteous because you pay so well, God. He is really loyal to me but knows he gets better inducements from you.'"

"Wow, I never saw that before," Harold exclaimed.

"So what does God do?"

"He gives Satan permission to have access to all Job possesses. He just can't kill Job."

"This is critical," I said: "Did God restrict what Satan could do to Job once God gave Satan permission to have access to Job? In other words, did God say Satan could only do harm, or was Job simply put in Satan's hands and Satan was free to do whatever Satan chose, short of killing Job?"

"Satan could do whatever he wanted, short of killing him."

"And what did Satan do?"

"He killed Job's children with a storm, destroyed his wealth and ruined his health."

"Absolutely," I said, "So we learn that Satan is the destroyer, not God. Satan was free to do whatever he wanted. In order to gain Job's loyalty himself, he could have had the other nations proclaim Job king and increase his wealth, territory and power, but he didn't. Why? Because Satan is the destroyer, not God. But notice how, in the story, the servants reported that the 'fire of God' fell and destroyed Job's possessions. Was God attacking Job or was this occurring by Satan's hand?"

"Satan was doing it, but God permitted it. Why would God allow it?"

"Perfect question, right on the money," I said. It was time to enlarge Harold's perspective, time for him to see his life from a higher vantage point. "Where did the book of Job begin?" I asked again.

"In heaven."

"And who was in attendance at that meeting?"

"God, his intelligent creatures and Satan."

"And when God made a judgment about Job being a trustworthy friend of his, Satan said, 'You're wrong, God. You're not telling the truth. Job is not who you claim he is. He doesn't love you and isn't faithful to you.' And here is the key to understanding what is really going on with Job: intelligent beings cannot read the secret intents of the hearts and minds of other intelligent beings. If they could, none of the angels would have been deceived by Lucifer in the first place. Therefore, if Satan gets Job to curse God, then Satan looks back to all those intelligent beings who are watching from heaven and says, 'See, I told you, God is wrong about Job, and he is wrong about me. You can't trust what God says!' Job was such a trusted friend of God that when God needed someone to step onto the witness stand of the universe to say what is right about God, Job was there. The issues in the book of Job were enormous, way beyond Job's individual pain and struggles.

"Job loved God and was willing to surrender himself to God's hands, to help God win the battle for hearts and minds of his intelligent children. And in Job 42:7-8, God commends Job twice for speaking 'the truth about me.' How many of God's children have been blessed by the history of Job?

"Harold," I pressed, "Have you considered the possibility that you are such a friend of God? Have you considered that God may be calling you to the witness stand of the universe to say what is right about him? That God may be saying to the universe, 'Have you considered my servant Harold? He is blameless and upright, a man who fears God and shuns evil.' And that Satan is attacking, trying to get you, like Job, to turn on God? No evil thing comes from God. God is the source of all good."

Harold was overwhelmed. He had never considered such a possibility. It was stupefying. He was struggling to get his mind around the implications. Could it really be this way? Could events in our individual lives actually be useful to God on a cosmic scale?

I read aloud 1 Corinthians 4:9, "For it seems to me that God has put us apostles on display at the end of the procession, like those condemned to die in the arena. We have been made a spectacle to the whole universe, to angels as well as to human beings."

"Harold," I asked, "could God be calling you to the arena, the theater of the universe to say what is right about him? Sometimes—rarely, in fact, but sometimes—tragic events and painful experiences happen because Satan is attacking God's friends, and we are witnessing to the entire universe our acceptance of God's grace and our loyalty to him."[1]

I continued, "Our confidence in God is based not on miracles but on the reality of who God is. God wins people to faith in him by the revelation of his trustworthiness as revealed ultimately in the life and death of Jesus Christ. Miracles can be counterfeited; the truth as revealed by Jesus cannot. The question is never about God's ability to perform miracles. The question is, do we know God well enough that our confidence will not be shaken when he doesn't miraculously intervene? Genuine faith is not having confidence that God can perform miracles but trusting him even when he—in our opinion—doesn't."

PRAYING FOR A MIRACLE

If, like many of my patients you have prayed for a miracle—a miracle of healing, of deliverance, of rejuvenation—yet God has not miraculously intervened, don't be disheartened, don't doubt your faith, and don't give in to discouragement. Instead, enlarge your perspective and consider the possibility that your faith may be of such quality, solidity and maturity that God knows you, like Job, will not be shaken out of trusting him. No matter what your hardship, let your unfailing trust in God shine out through the darkness of sin's oppressive assault, and declare before the entire universe that God is worthy of your trust and you will not be shaken from him. Miraculous intervention or not, God is worthy of your trust![2]

This is how Harold enlarged his perspective. He accepted the truth that genuine faith does not mean God will miraculously intervene. Genuine faith is trusting God not to intervene if he has other purposes for your life. Initially, Harold didn't know what God's purpose was in not healing him, but Harold's despair lifted, his fear resolved, his doubts disappeared, even though his cancer remained.

From then on, as he went to treatment, he went with a smile on his face. Rather than focusing on himself and his tragic situation, he instead allowed God's love to flow through him to others. He inquired about the nurses: their lives, families and struggles. He prayed with them, encouraged them and sought to share God's love wherever he went. He spent time with his family, not in depression, but living, loving and encouraging them. His life had become a bright shining ray of godly love in the midst of a dark and dying world.

God did not *bring* cancer on Harold. But when the cancer developed, God chose not to intervene to heal the cancer, because God brings good out of evil when we trust him. Before he died, Harold was privileged to see the answer to his question, "Why me, Lord?" Two of Harold's siblings had walked away from God some years before. They were successful in business, wealthy and affluent, but had no time for God in their lives. They were living for the world and Harold had worried for their souls. He had spent years praying for them, for their redemption, often praying, "Use me, Father, to reach my brother and sister for your kingdom, if it be your will." It was this prayer that God answered.

When Harold's siblings saw his life slowly ebb away and observed his persistent joy, his steadfast happiness, his determined love for others, their hearts were convicted. They saw that Harold possessed something that all the money in the world couldn't buy—genuine peace. They realized their lives were the ones that needed healing. They returned to God, were rebaptized and rededicated their lives to the Lord, and are now faithful and active members in their church. Truly, Harold had been called to the arena to be a spectacle of God's love to others, perhaps even to angels.

Shortly before he died, Harold told me, "God is so amazing. When cancer assaulted me, God took this evil and worked his grace through me as the way to reach my brother and sister for his kingdom. If that is what it took to reach them, I am privileged to do it. Surely, 'in all things God works for the good of those who love him, who have been called according to his purpose' [Rom 8:28]. I may have had my life shortened by a few decades here on earth, but if it results in their eternal salvation, then I will have an eternity to rejoice with them and with the rest of my family—in a world free from all sin, disease and heartache."

Harold is no longer with us on this earth, but his witness remains, his memory remains, and the lesson he gave us remains. By stepping back and taking a larger view, Harold was able to work with God to bring good out of evil. It is when we stop running from fear, embrace the truth, and love others more than ourselves that God's healing love overrules evil and brings forth good.

The Judgment of God

Friendship consists in forgetting what one gives,
and remembering what one receives.

ALEXANDRE DUMAS PÈRE

WHEN I WAS A CHILD, my favorite part of church was children's story time. Each week before the sermon, the children would rush to the front of the church, reverently of course, while the pianist played "Jesus Loves the Little Children." Every story was something new. At different times the storyteller brought puppies, a snakeskin, balloons and strange-looking masks from Africa. Perhaps the cutest was the time we got to pet ducklings. I loved children's story time, but there was one tale that haunted me for years.

The saga began with a little boy who stole a cookie. As the narrative unfolded, an angel appeared onstage—someone dressed in a white robe with long blonde hair, glittered face, golden halo and white wings, and holding a golden clipboard and pen. My eyes grew wide as I watched the angel almost float across the stage. As the storyteller described various infractions—talking back to mommy, fighting over a toy or making an ugly face—the angel dutifully wrote on the clipboard.

We were told that God sends his recording angels to follow us everywhere we go and faithfully write down every sin we commit in heaven's record books. Only by confessing our sins and asking Jesus to forgive could the sins be erased from those heavenly ledgers. If we didn't ask Jesus to forgive, our sins would remain in the books and, at judgment, when God saw them, he would punish accordingly.

I experienced so many restless nights, so many nightmares because of that story. Most alarming of all, I found myself becoming afraid of God. I worried I might forget to confess a sin and not get it erased. In my imagination I could see that angel with the golden clipboard following me around, hounding my every step, and I didn't like it. I didn't feel God's love as much as I felt his scrutiny. I didn't want to make mistakes, so I worked hard to do everything right. I paid my tithe, read my Bible, prayed three times a day and imagined all the good things I did were being recorded by the angel and hoped it counted for something. But I didn't have peace. All my actions were based on fear of punishment, not love for God and my fellow human beings, for love does not flow where lies about God are retained.

POLICEMAN IN THE SKY

A friend recently told me of an encounter she had with a pastor at a local bookstore. The pastor was cautioning her about the impact that my book *Could It Be This Simple?* was having on members of his congregation. He was not pleased because his message was very different from mine. Then he said, pointing upward, "God is the Great Policeman in the sky. He watches for any violations of his law and enforces justly the penalties for disobedience."

Have you ever been driving along and had a police car pull in behind you? How did you feel? And what if the police officer followed you closely for several miles—did the apprehension build?

Did you start to feel scrutinized, to worry that he or she was watching you, waiting for some mistake that would warrant pulling you over and ticketing you? Did you even start thinking back over the past few years, wondering if there was some infraction that slipped by, some parking ticket you hadn't paid, some forgotten error in judgment that had taken place while you were behind the wheel—an error unnoticed by you but dutifully observed by a member of law enforcement?

Sadly, many people have accepted this twisted perspective about God. Now, it's not all bad news to those who hold such a view. They are quick to remind us not to be afraid of what God might see us do because, when we accept Jesus, he stands between us and the Father and functions like a heavenly radar-jammer, his atoning blood distorting the vengeful Father's ability to see our sins!

For me, it was only once I began to see God through the life of Jesus that my misconception of him vanished and my fear faded away. I saw God in a new light. I thought of the riders persevering through the grueling Tour de France. A car follows each team throughout the course. If one should fall, members of his team are there to quickly assist, bandage any wound, repair damage to his bike and get him back on his way. Likewise, God has his agencies following us throughout our lives, but for what purpose? Always to bandage our wounds, repair our broken lives and put us back on the path to eternal life.

As I have taught these truths, both in writing and behind the pulpit, I have found that many Christians are held in bondage by fear of facing the record of their sins, just as I had been. One of my greatest joys in life is sharing truth that sets people free.

THE HEAVENLY RECORDS

Helen possesses such a sharp mind. Having her in my weekly Bible study class is a real privilege. She is one of those people who seems to have a thousand questions and isn't afraid to ask.

One day after class we had the following conversation.

"Dr. Jennings, I remember you said that one of the misunderstandings with which we sometimes struggle is the idea that Jesus is
in heaven erasing sins out of the heavenly record books. I think you
said he isn't doing that, but if he is not erasing the record of sins, then
how do we understand these Bible verses?"

> I, even I, am he who blots out
>   your transgressions, for my own sake,
>   and remembers your sins no more. (Is 43:25)

And,

> For I will forgive their wickedness
>   and will remember their sins no more. (Heb 8:12)

"Good for you," I said. "I am so glad you are studying and inquiring for yourself. How have you heard these verses explained in
the past?"

"When we confess our sins, God erases them from the record
books of heaven and then, at the judgment, the saved don't have to
face the record of their sins," Helen said.

"That's what I was taught as well," I told her. "But does either of
the verses actually say sin is being blotted out of record books? In
fact, are record books mentioned at all?"

"Huh, no, I hadn't noticed that before," she replied slowly. "But
in Revelation it says, 'And I saw the dead, great and small, standing
before the throne, and books were opened. Another book was
opened, which is the book of life. The dead were judged according
to what they had done as recorded in the books' [Rev 20:12]. If God
is not blotting sins out of the record books of heaven, then what is it
talking about?"

"Hold on," I cautioned with a smile, "let's not get ahead of ourselves. Let's first explore another assumption that underpins the
idea of erasing sins from record books. Have you been taught that
God has recording angels keeping track of all our sins, and one day

we will face those sins in the judgment—unless of course we confess them and ask forgiveness, and then Jesus or God erases them from the record?"

"Yes, that is exactly how I was taught."

"Me too. But as I read the Bible through several times, some things started to not add up using that popular perspective. Do you believe, as the Bible teaches, that God is love?"

"Now more than ever."

"Notice what the Bible says about love: 'Love is patient, love is kind. It does not envy, it does not boast, it is not proud. It does not dishonor others, it is not self-seeking, it is not easily angered,' and"—I paused—"'it keeps no record of wrongs' [1 Cor 13:4-5, emphasis mine]. If love keeps no record of wrongs, and God is love, does it make sense that God is keeping a record of all our wrongs in order to judge or punish us?"

Before she could answer I continued, "Listen to this incredible passage: 'Therefore, if anyone is in Christ, he is a new creation; the old has gone, the new has come! All this is from God, who reconciled us to himself through Christ and gave us the ministry of reconciliation: that God was reconciling the world to himself in Christ, *not counting men's sins against them*. And he has committed to us the message of reconciliation' (2 Cor 5:17-19 NIV 1984, emphasis mine). If God is working, through Christ, to reconcile us to himself, to heal us and make us right with him again, if he is not counting our sins against us, then does it make sense that he is keeping a record of our sins in order to punish us?"

"No," my friend stated, "but doesn't he have to keep track of our sins in order to be fair?"

"You can be sure that God is always fair. But don't we need to bring harmony to how we understand all these passages? How is it that the Bible speaks of record books in heaven, God blotting out our sin, but also of love not keeping record of our wrongs? How do all these ideas fit together so that all are equally true?"

"Good question," she mumbled.

"When I was in my fourth year of medical school, I did a rotation in the ER. One day there was a helicopter crash at the local airport that left six people seriously injured. They were rushed to our hospital, where we worked furiously to save them. There was one woman I will never forget. She arrived with both femurs—the large bones in her thighs—fractured, a fractured pelvis and broken ribs. When she was wheeled in, she was awake, oriented and aware of her situation. The broken bones in her pelvis and upper legs caused severe bleeding into the tissues of her thighs that, if left unresolved, would result in her death. She needed a blood transfusion and emergency surgery to save her life. With this treatment the likelihood of survival was very high. Without treatment she would most certainly die. But this woman was a Jehovah's Witness, and she believed blood transfusions are forbidden by God. Therefore, she refused the treatment.

"As her life was slowly ebbing away, we appealed to her. We knew we could save her if she would only allow us, if she would accept a blood transfusion, so we began to plead with her. The nurses begged, the doctors implored, and we lowly medical students appealed to her, but she remained resolute. The hospital chaplain reasoned and prayed with her and, eventually, even the hospital administrator and staff lawyer earnestly implored her to let us save her, but she still refused. From the time she rejected the blood transfusion until she lost consciousness, some member of the hospital team was by her side, trying to get her to accept our life-saving treatment. But once she lost consciousness, no one could plead with her anymore.

"Not only did the treatment team reason with this woman, trying to convince her to let us heal her, but we also intervened with her life-threatening injuries. We worked to hold death at bay. We gave volume enhancers called IV fluids, used blood recyclers (she would accept her own blood) and applied pneumatic-pressure devices, all designed to stop the blood loss and prevent death's approach. But, sadly, while every other victim of that crash survived, this woman died."

My friend Helen sat riveted, so I continued, "Now, if her family brought a lawsuit against the doctors, nurses and hospital for failing to save this lady, they'd claim: 'They saved everyone else on that helicopter but let our mother die. They aren't compassionate. They aren't loving. They don't care equally for all people. They're biased; they play favorites. Some people they save and some they don't.' What then would come into evidence?"

"The medical records!" Helen exclaimed.

"Absolutely! And would the records be brought into evidence in order to judge and punish this lady, or would the records be brought into evidence to defend the health-care team?"

"To defend the health-care team." Helen paused as a new thought raced through her mind. Then she said, "Are you telling me that the records are being kept to defend God?"

In reply I directed her to what Paul said in Romans 3:4, speaking about God. I read it in three different translations of Scripture so there could be no confusion, and I emphasized what I believe to be the important portions as they related to our conversation:

God must be true, even though all human beings are liars. As the scripture says,
  "You must be shown to be right when you speak;
    you must win your case when you are being tried." (GNT)

Let God be true, but every man a liar; as it is written, That thou mightest be justified in thy sayings, and *mightest overcome when thou art judged.* (KJV)

Let God be found true though every man be found a liar, as it is written,
  "That You may be justified in Your words,
    And prevail when You are judged." (ESV)

"Contrary to what so many think," I told Helen, "the heavenly records are like detailed medical records, accurately recording our condition, the treatments offered and our responses. If someone makes allegations against a doctor, medical records are there to defend him, not to accuse, embarrass or punish the patient. In the same way, we can bring harmony to the Scripture by understanding that our God of love doesn't keep track of our sins in order to punish us; he keeps records in order to document that he did everything he could to save and heal every one of us. These records will demonstrate that if anyone is lost, it is because they refused his treatment, not because of some failure on God's part. While love keeps no record of wrongs, we still have records in heaven, 'medical' records documenting the facts of each case, demonstrating what an awesome God we have, demonstrating how long God and his agencies pled with each and every sinner lost."

After several minutes of reflection Helen brought up another point. "But what about the blotting out of our sins? How do we fit in those texts?"

"Where does sin occur? In record books or in hearts and minds of intelligent beings?"

"In us, in our hearts and minds," she said.

"Then, from where does God want to blot out sin? From the recorded history of the universe, or from the hearts, minds and characters of his children? The Bible leaves no doubt as to where God is working to remove sin."

> For he [Christ] will be like a refiner's fire or a launderer's soap. He will sit as a refiner and purifier of silver; *he will purify the Levites* and refine them like gold and silver. (Mal 3:2-3, emphasis mine)

"God is working to remove sinfulness from our hearts and minds, to cleanse and purify us. Think back on one of the very passages you cited about God not remembering our sins anymore. What happens before God says he won't remember our sins?"

This is the covenant that I will make with the house of Israel
after those days, says the Lord: I will put my laws in their minds,
and write them on their hearts, and I will be their God, and
they shall be my people. And they shall not teach one another
or say to each other, "Know the Lord," for they shall all know
me, from the least of them to the greatest. For I will be merciful
toward their iniquities, and I will remember their sins no more.
(Heb 8:10-12 NRSV)

"He is healing our hearts?" Helen asked.

"God is blotting sinfulness from the hearts and minds of his
people. He is restoring his law of love into the inmost being. Just as
there is no reason for a doctor to think about sickness once we are
well, there is no reason for God to think about or remember our
sinfulness once we are perfectly restored to his original ideal."

After thinking silently for several minutes, Helen told me the
picture of God I shared sounded beautiful, but it was so different
from what she had been taught her entire life that she would have to
study more on her own.

RECORDS AND THE BRAIN

Do our beliefs about such things as records in heaven really matter?
Beliefs—such as God being a great policeman in the sky, a cosmic
inquisitor, a being who watches to mete out proper punishment—
incite fear and activate the amygdala (fear circuit). The constantly
active amygdala activates the body's immune system, the specialized
white blood cells called macrophages. Why? Because our immune
system is to our body what our National Guard is to our nation. It
protects us from invasion, and when the alarm fires, it signals the
immune system to get ready for invasion.

Imagine you are walking in the Smoky Mountain National Park
and, rounding a corner, you come face to face with a black bear. Not
only do you instantly become alert but, when your "alarm" fires,

your body prepares for "fight or flight." In this emergency situation, if you fight the bear and survive, it is likely that your skin will be breached and an invasion of microscopic pathogens will occur. With every emergency, it's like your brain putting your body on DEFCON 2: prepare for invasion.

Every time the "alarm" fires, it primes the body's immune system to prepare for attack. The body has two types of immunity, acquired and innate. Acquired immunity is what we exploit with vaccines. When we give a vaccine, we introduce antigens of the harmful enemy invaders into the body. Antigens are the identifying markers unique to each organism, analogous to an enemy's flag. When we give the vaccine, our immune system identifies the enemy by its flag (antigen) and creates antibodies specific for that invader. The antibodies will then function as snipers. They sit and wait for that one particular enemy invader and will kill it and only it.

This is not the immunity we activate when confronted by a bear. The body in emergency mode doesn't have time to make antibodies, so under stress the body activates the innate immunity. This is analogous to grabbing a sawed-off shotgun under the bed during a home invasion. It is dark, you hear commotion and threat, you point the gun and blast a wide radius. You get the invader, but you also damage the house. The house in our story is the body.

When the alarm (amygdala) fires, it activates macrophages, which begin releasing inflammatory cytokines. These cytokines (such as interleuken-1, interleuken-6 and tumor-necrosis factor) are analogous to our shotgun pellets, designed to destroy the enemy, but just like the pellets, these inflammatory factors also wreak havoc throughout the "house" (body).

Under chronic activation (stress), the cytokines damage the neurons that tell the brain, "Enough stress hormones have been released so don't call for any more." The glucocorticoid receptors on our hippocampal neurons are attacked, and we lose the feedback inhibition on the 911 operator (hypothalamus). The 911 operator then begins calling for more stress hormones. This causes further elevation in blood glucose, heart rate and blood pressure, as well as increasing other effects of stress.

Simultaneously, the cytokines damage insulin receptors in the body, making it harder for the body to use glucose. The combined effect of prolonged activation of this stress cascade is increased risk of type 2 diabetes, obesity, elevated cholesterol and triglycerides, bone loss, heart attacks, strokes, ulcers, infections and inflammatory disorders. The cytokines also increase the perception of pain and interfere with brain neurotransmitters, so a person in chronic stress will typically experience decreased energy, motivation, impaired concentration, decreased appetite, aches and pains, and sleep disturbance.[1]

Fear-inducing beliefs really do damage us, and our individual beliefs are building blocks forming the ultimate picture we hold about God. The more erroneous blocks (individual doctrinal beliefs), the more distorted our picture. The greater the distortion about God, the more activation of the brain's fear circuits, and the farther we move from God's healing plan. Yes, our beliefs about God really do matter.

13

In the Brain of Christ

I know men and I tell you that Jesus Christ
is no mere man. Between Him and every other person
in the world there is no possible term of comparison. Alexander,
Caesar, Charlemagne, and I have founded empires. But on
what did we rest the creation of our genius? Upon force.
Jesus Christ founded His empire upon love; and at
this hour millions of men would die for Him.

NAPOLEON BONAPARTE

ANISSA AYALA WAS AFRAID. She didn't like going to the doctor and hated needles even more, so she hid the stomach cramps, numbing aches, persistent pains and mysterious lumps from her parents. She suffered for weeks until, on Easter Sunday 1988, the agony became too great and she realized she needed help.

Lab tests were performed and she was given the grim diagnosis of chronic myelogenous leukemia. Without a bone marrow transplant, she would be dead in three to five years.[1]

Immediately her family was tested. Mother, Mary, 43; father, Abe, 45; and, brother, Airon, 19, all failed to be suitable donor matches. The National Bone Marrow Donor Registry was checked but, unfortunately, there were no matches.[2]

Abe and Mary were desperate. What could they do? Their precious daughter was dying! Mary and Abe decided to try to have another child, hoping they could capitalize on the one-in-four chance of a sibling match. This would not be easy. Not only was age against them, but Abe would need to have his vasectomy, performed sixteen years earlier, reversed.

Soon word spread of what the Ayalas were planning. Critics began to mount, questioning the ethics and morals of bringing a child into the world to be a tissue donor. But Mary and Abe didn't care what the critics said. They had a child to save.

Abe had the vasectomy reversed and, within six months, Mary became pregnant. As the pregnancy progressed, tissue sampling was performed and they rejoiced to discover their unborn child was a tissue match. Fourteen months after Anissa's little sister, Marissa Eve, was born, a bone marrow transplant was performed, saving Anissa's life.

We rejoice to read of love's triumph in the Ayala family. But their saga also offers powerful insights into our terminal condition and God's plan of salvation. Why did Mary and Abe bring Marissa into the world? Why did this innocent baby have to shed its blood? Because it was needed in order to heal and save their other girl. And, in the face of critics, Abe said, "We thought we were going to lose a daughter and now we have two."[3]

IT'S IN THE BLOOD

Leukemia is cancer of the blood. And cancer is caused by cells that have lost self-control, cells that replicate out of control, cells that no longer operate in harmony with their design. Cancer always leads to death unless some intervention, some intercession, is performed in order to put the cancer into remission. Unless something is done to change the cancerous cells back to their precancerous healthy state, death is sure to follow. Without the shedding of Marissa's blood, there could be no remission of Anissa's leukemia.

Without the shedding of Christ's blood, there is no remission of sin (Heb 9:22). Without the victory of Jesus at the cross we could not be changed back into our original, pre-selfish, loving, God-like state—the way humankind emerged from the hand and breath of God in Eden.

No one knows why Anissa got leukemia, but what if at age five she disobeyed her father's command to never play with the pesticides in the garage and the leukemia was determined to be a direct result of disobedience and exposure to this toxin? If that were the case, would justice require that her father let her die? Or worse yet, would justice require her father kill her to punish her for her disobedience? Exactly what would justice require her father to do if that justice was based on the law of love?

What if her father had said, "In the day you drink the pesticide, you will surely die"? If he had said those words, would her father need to let her die in order to be just? If her father did warn her, "In the day you drink the pesticides, you will surely die," would he be saying it as a threat or as a warning to protect?

And once she had this terminal condition, what must transpire in order to be just, in order not to violate the laws of health? The cancer must be sent into remission. The unhealthy, deformed cells must *remit*. And what is the only way to make that happen? With a remedy and a cure!

Why did God say to Adam, "In the day you eat this fruit, you will die"? Because God would be forced to kill him? Or because humankind would thus deviate from the law of love, the law of life, and without intervention, the only consequence would be ruin and death? Once our first parents infected themselves with this terminal condition, what was needed? A remedy and a cure. That cure was born as a baby in Bethlehem.

LOVE RISKS BEING MISUNDERSTOOD IN ORDER TO SAVE

As I have presented these ideas from place to place, I've met individuals who don't like this view. They struggle with this truth because of statements in the Bible in which God seems to be saying, "I'm mad. I'm angry. And in my wrath, I'm going to kill!"

> The city of murderers is doomed! *I myself will pile up the firewood.* Bring more wood! Fan the flames! Cook the meat! Boil away the broth! Burn up the bones! Now set the empty bronze pot on the coals and let it get red-hot. . . . You will not be pure again until you have felt the full force of my anger. I, the LORD, have spoken. The time has come for me to act. I will not ignore your sins or show pity or be merciful. You will be punished for what you have done. (Ezek 24:9-11, 13-14 GNT, emphasis mine)

At first glance this text sounds terrifying. I remember how I used to struggle with passages like this, always afraid that God was waiting to get me—and get me good—if I slipped up. But I realized my misunderstandings about God occurred only because I never asked the right questions when reading these difficult texts. The question is not whether God spoke these words through his prophet, for I am confident he did. The important question is: What actually happened *after* he spoke these words?

Did God use his power to destroy those about whom he spoke such terrifying words? Or did their rebellion separate them from his protection, thus resulting in their destruction?

The children of Israel refused to follow God, his methods and principles. But God did not hurt them. Instead, he set them free. He gave them what they chose—a life separated from him. He stopped interceding on their behalf. He removed his protective hand at their insistence, and before long, here came the Babylonians who, in true Babylonian style, destroyed their city. It was the Babylonians, not God, who delivered the destructive punch.

This letting go by God, this setting free to reap the consequences of our own persistent, rebellious choices, is what the Bible calls "God's wrath." Paul tells us the "wrath" of God occurs because of persistently rejecting God, refusing the knowledge of him and preferring our own way over God's. Then Paul states three times that, in the first century after Christ, the unruly experienced God's wrath when God "gave them over" to the consequences of their own choices (Rom 1:18-32).

I am not the first to draw such a conclusion:

The human condition, which Paul describes in Romans 1:18-32, is not something caused by God. The phrase "revealed from heaven" (where "heaven" is a typical Jewish substitute word for "God") does not depict some kind of divine intervention, but rather the *inevitability of human debasement* which results when God's will, built into the created order, is violated. Since the created order has its origin in God, Paul can say that the wrath of God is now (constantly) being revealed "from heaven." It is revealed in the fact that the rejection of God's truth (Rom 1:18-20), that is, the truth about God's nature and will, leads to futile thinking (Rom 1.21-22), idolatry (Rom 1:23), perversion of God-intended sexuality (Rom 1:24-27) and relational-moral brokenness (Rom 1:28-32). [Scriptural emphasis theirs.]

The expression "God gave them over" (or "handed them over"), which appears three times in this passage (Rom 1:24, 26, 28), supports the idea that the sinful perversion of human existence, though resulting from human decisions, is to be understood ultimately as God's punishment which we, in freedom, bring upon ourselves.

In light of these reflections, the common notion that God punishes or blesses in direct proportion to our sinful or good deeds cannot be maintained. . . . God loves us with an everlasting love. But the rejection of that love separates us from its life-giving power. The result is disintegration and death.[4]

Jesus, who became sin for us, experienced God's "wrath" at the cross and cried out, "My God, my God, why have you forsaken me?"—not "Why are you killing me?" (Mt 27:46). All through the Bible, the story is the same.

In Deuteronomy God's wrath is threatened: "For a fire will be kindled by my wrath, one that burns down to the realm of the dead below. It will devour the earth and its harvests and set afire the foundations of the mountains. I will heap calamities on them and spend my arrows against them" (Deut 32:22-23). But God says the wise will understand what his wrath really is: "If only they were wise and would understand this and discern what their end will be! How could one man chase a thousand, or two put ten thousand to flight, unless their Rock had sold them, *unless the* LORD *had given them up?*" (Deut 32:29-30, emphasis mine).

LOVE CANNOT BE FORCED

The wise understand that love cannot be forced, only freely given. The discerning realize that the angriest, most wrathful act Love can take is to let the object of his love go. Again, God makes plain that his anger or wrath is letting go. "When that happens, I will become angry with them; *I will abandon them,* and they will be destroyed. Many terrible disasters will come upon them, and then they will realize that these things are happening to them because *I, their God, am no longer with them*" (Deut 31:17 GNT, emphasis mine).

But why would God speak in such threatening language through Ezekiel if it was the Babylonians and not him that actually burned the city?

When our children are in danger, when they will not listen, do we as loving parents raise our voices to warn and protect? "The people of Israel are as stubborn as mules. How can I feed them like lambs in a meadow?" (Hos 4:16 GNT). God hates to speak such harsh words, but the God of love risks all in order to save his children.

Imagine you have a ten-year-old son, and he is a stubborn, unruly and difficult child. He doesn't listen to your instructions. When you tell him to pick up his clothes, he argues. When you tell him to turn off the television, he ignores you. He won't complete his chores without your constant threats.

One day your family is visiting a national park with steep canyon walls. Your son is playing Frisbee and running directly toward the cliff. He is too far away to reach, so you shout for him to stop. But your child is unruly: he doesn't listen but keeps running toward the cliff. What would you do? As he nears the precipice, would you threaten? "If you don't stop right now, I am going to beat your bottom raw!" If your child didn't stop and went over the cliff, would you climb down, take off your belt and beat him? Would you get out a rifle and shoot your child as he fell toward the rocks below in order to punish him for his disobedience? Do you have to inflict any suffering on your child in order to be "just"? Of course not. But violations of the law—including the law of gravity—result in death. If your child wouldn't stop, there would be nothing for you to do except mourn.

That is exactly how it is with God and us. Listen to his pleading words: "How can I give you up, Israel? How can I abandon you? . . . My heart will not let me do it! My love for you is too strong" (Hos 11:8 GNT). "Jerusalem, Jerusalem, you who kill the prophets and stone those sent to you, how often I have longed to gather your children together, as a hen gathers her chicks under her wings, and you were not willing" (Mt 23:37). As your willful, headstrong, irresponsible son falls to his death, like God, you would cry out, "My son, my son, how I have longed to protect you, to keep you safe, but you were stubborn like a mule and wouldn't listen."

We are all sick and dying, and we all need real healing and real transformation in our lives. That baby in Bethlehem is our remedy. He came to do that which no human could do for himself: to heal our condition, all within the bounds of God's eternal law of love.

CAVEATS ABOUT ATONEMENT

The study of what Christ accomplished at the cross will occupy our minds throughout eternity. Into an everlasting future, our hearts will rejoice as new insights about what Christ accomplished are understood. Therefore, while it is my intention to describe specific achievements accomplished by Christ, I do not presume to present the final word on the atonement but a progressive word that I hope others will grasp and continue to unfold.

I purposely focus our view of Christ's achievements within his humanity, specifically his human brain. I mean to be precise and clear, describing an explicit procurement achieved by Christ through the exercise of his human brain. The key to understanding Christ's mission to earth, his victory at the cross, hinges on rightly understanding God's law of love as the design template on which life is constructed. A review of chapter 1 might be helpful at this point.

Regardless of whether you value this perspective, or prefer a different understanding (as Christianity has historically held a variety of atonement models),[5] when it comes to our salvation it is not necessary to understand the atonement to benefit from it. All that is necessary is to surrender in trust to God.

Imagine a patient is dying with a terminal condition. If there is a cure for his condition, the only requirement that the patient must meet in order to be healed is that he "trust" the doctor by following the treatment protocol. The patient does not have to understand how the treatment works. He does not have to understand how the treatment was developed. All the patient has to do is trust the doctor, take the prescription, and if the doctor has a remedy that cures, the patient will be healed. Likewise, sinners don't have to understand anything about how Christ achieves our salvation in order to be saved, but we do have to trust God and accept his treatment in order to benefit from all that Christ has done.

However, from the doctor's perspective, things are very different. He or she must properly diagnose the problem, procure a remedy (which generally requires understanding how it is developed and should be applied) and provide evidence of his or her trustworthiness in order for the remedy to be accepted by the patient.

When the requirements of the atonement are stated as only needing to reestablish trust, it seems this is true regarding the vantage point of the sinner. All we need, in order to be saved/healed, is to have trust reestablished in the one who gave us life. We don't have to understand how God through Christ achieved our salvation; we don't have to understand how the Holy Spirit administers what Christ accomplished into our lives; but we *do* have to trust God and follow his directions.

But, as we become understanding friends of God, we begin to contemplate what God had to accomplish in order to fix the damage that sin caused. As a physician I take seriously Jesus' invitation to understand what he has done and is doing (Jn 15:15). I seek, as far as a finite mind can, to understand salvation from his vantage point. This takes us beyond just trusting our Great Physician to genuinely understanding.

WHY JESUS HAD TO DIE

Lies believed by Adam and Eve broke the circle of love and trust, and they resulted in humanity being changed from beings living in harmony with the law of love to beings operating on fear and selfishness. Jesus died to reverse all of this. The Bible says he gave his life to "destroy" Satan, death and the devil's work (2 Tim 1:9-10; Heb 2:14; 1 Jn 3:8).

In order to do this, Jesus had to accomplish two goals. First, he had to reveal the truth about God in order to destroy Satan's lies and win us back to trust. And second, he had to put the law of love back into the human species. His goal was to reconnect humanity with the circle of life. He accomplished this by becoming the vehicle, conduit, connecting link, avenue through which God's love could flow back into humankind.

Imagine you have bacterial endocarditis—an infection of the interior of the heart. Without a remedy, this is a terminal condition. A man comes to you claiming to have a substance that will cure you and wants to inject you with it. You are an American and his name is Osama bin Laden. Would you let him inject you? Why not? Because you don't trust him. It doesn't matter whether he has a remedy or not; if there is no trust we won't take the remedy and thus won't get well. Christ had to reveal the truth to destroy the lies of Satan and win us back to trust—step one of his mission. But he had to do more.

What if you have a loving father who happens to be a physician, and you trust him completely, but he has no remedy for endocarditis. Will your trust in your father get you well? No. Trust only works when there actually is a remedy. We are not saved by faith or trust. We are saved by grace, which is God's work of restoring love in us when we trust him. It takes both—the restoration of trust and a real remedy—to bring about healing.

Satan tried to obstruct God at both places. He worked to prevent Christ from coming as a human and procuring a real remedy. But, as we explored in chapter 4, God acted to thwart Satan and keep open the channel for the Messiah to come. Evil forces tried to have baby Jesus killed before he could complete his mission, before Jesus lived out perfect love in human form. God, again, intervened to stop the enemy of good. God knew that the *mere* shedding of his son's innocent blood was not what was needed to save humankind, so he protected the baby Jesus from Satan's assault until Jesus completed his mission years later.

Satan failed to shut the avenue. He failed to kill the baby Jesus, and he failed in his temptations of Christ. Jesus Christ defeated Satan and has procured a real remedy to heal humanity. No matter how one describes the atonement, no matter how we comprehend it, Jesus has achieved what is necessary for our salvation. Therefore, Satan's only remaining strategy is to tell lies about God, lies that, when believed, prevent us from trusting him. For if we don't trust God, we won't accept his treatment.

HOW JESUS ACHIEVED OUR REMEDY

Jesus Christ is a unique being in the history of the universe. Adam was made from dust, and God breathed into his nostrils the breath of life and he became a living being; Eve was taken from the side of sinless Adam. You and I did not come into the world this way; we were born from a sinful mother and a sinful father (Ps 51:5). Amazingly, Jesus' incarnation did not occur in either of these ways.

His humanity was not created out of the dust like Adam's or taken from the side of a sinless human being, like Eve's; nor was Jesus born of both a sinful mother and sinful father like you and I. Jesus was unique. He was born of a sinful mother, born of a woman under the law of sin and death (Rom 8:2; Gal 4:4). But his Father is God. The Holy Spirit came upon a sinful woman to form Jesus' humanity (Mt 1:18). Jesus joined his divinity to our humanity. Why? To destroy fear and selfishness and perfectly restore the law of love back into the human species.

Jesus Christ is the member of the human family in whom the law of love was never broken! Jesus is the one human being whose brain loved perfectly. In Jesus Christ the two antagonistic principles warred it out—love others or promote self. Jesus came to crush the serpent's head. As soon as Jesus was baptized and "full of the Holy Spirit," he was led by the Spirit to the wilderness (Lk 4:1), in order to be tempted by the devil so that he might overcome fear and selfishness with love—all within his human brain.

Satan came at him with both barrels blazing. "If you are the Son of God, turn this stone into bread"—*save* yourself. "If you are the Son of God, jump off this tower"—*prove* yourself. "If you are the Son of God, bow down to me"—*save* yourself.

Jesus was "tempted in every way, just as we are—yet he did not sin" (Heb 4:15). And remember, each one of us "is tempted when, by his own evil desire, he is dragged away and enticed" (Jas 1:14 NIV 1984). We experience the constant, internal temptation to act in self-interest, to protect self—and Jesus took this sick condition on himself. He experienced the full force of evil's onslaught, but he overcame it by the power of self-sacrificing love. Jesus became our substitute in that he took our "sinfulness," our "terminal condition," our "iniquity," our "infirmity" (Is 53:4) on himself in order to cure, heal and restore humankind back into God's original ideal. He became "sin for us, so that in him we might become the righteousness of God" (2 Cor 5:21). He took our sick condition and cured it!

POWERFUL EMOTIONS

In Gethsemane, Jesus' humanity was overwhelmed with anguish. He was tempted with powerful emotions, so strong that he said he was nearing death. And, according to Jesus' own testimony, what did the powerful emotions tempt him to do? Save himself (Mt 26:36-42)! But with each temptation Jesus chose to give himself in love. Every time the temptation to act in self-interest assaulted him, he overcame by loving others and giving of himself perfectly. Jesus said, "No one takes it [my life] from me, but I lay it down of my own accord. I have authority to lay it down and authority to take it up again. This command I received from my Father" (Jn 10:18). In Jesus Christ the law of love destroyed the law of sin and death.

"For whoever wants to save his life will lose it, but whoever loses their life for me will find it" (Mt 16:25). When Jesus refused to use his power to save himself but instead offered himself freely, he destroyed death (selfishness is the basis of death) and brought life and immortality to light (2 Tim 1:9-10). Therefore he rose again, still partaking of humanity, but with a humanity that he had purified, cleansed and perfectly re-created to God's original design. His resurrection was the natural result, the inevitable outcome, of destroying the infection of selfishness and restoring God's law of life—the law of love—back into humanity. "The law of the Lord is perfect, reviving the soul" (Ps 19:7 NIV 1984).

Why did he have to die? If at any point along death's approach Christ would have used his power to stop it from consuming him, who would he have saved? Self! The only way to destroy selfishness was by perfect self-sacrificing love. Christ restored the law of life into humanity by giving himself freely in love.

Thus "once made perfect, he became the source of eternal salvation for all who obey him" (Heb 5:9). He is our remedy, our Savior, the God-man through whom God's very nature of love flows back into humanity again. Christ did what no other being could do. He revealed the truth about God to win us to trust; but more than that, he became our substitute by taking our condition on himself in order to cure, fix and heal humanity in his own person. In other words, he perfected humanity! He achieved what Adam was created to become.

It is because of Christ's victory, because of his achievement, that all who trust him will be infused with his Holy Spirit, the one who takes all Christ has achieved and reproduces it in us. Through Christ we are healed to live eternally with him!

Jesus said, "I tell you the truth: It is for your good that I am going away. Unless I go away, the Counselor will not come to you; but if I go, I will send him to you. . . . I have much more to say to you, more than you can now bear. But when he, the Spirit of truth, comes, he will guide you into all truth. He will not speak on his own; he will speak only what he hears, and he will tell you what is yet to come. He will glorify me by *taking what is mine and making it known to you.* All that belongs to the Father is mine. That is why I said the Spirit *will take what is mine and make it known to you*" (Jn 16:7, 12-15 NIV 1984, emphasis mine).

What is Christ's that we need? A pure heart and right spirit, a perfect character of love. When we trust him, he pours his love into our hearts (Rom 5:5). God is love; therefore, when he pours his love into our hearts he is actually pouring himself into our hearts (1 Jn 4:8). His perfect character of love is created within us by the indwelling Spirit; it is no longer I who lives but Christ who lives in me (Gal 2:20). We literally become partakers of God's divine nature of love (2 Pet 1:4). We are restored back to "at-one-ment" with God.

What I am saying is this: God possesses a perfect divine nature; angels in heaven possess perfect angelic natures, beings on other worlds (assuming they exist) are in possession of perfect natures of their order—but, after Adam's sin and before Christ's victory, there was no perfect human nature. Christ came to fix this, to within the human species, restore perfection of character, to rewrite God's law of love into humanity. Divinity can create a new order/species anytime divinity chooses—but because of the nature of love and liberty, humanity, once defective, could only be cured by the exercise of human choice. No human, descended from Adam, could accomplish this, but Christ, uniting his divinity with our humanity did this work. In order to cure this creation, a human being had to exercise trust in God. A human being had to reject the lies and temptations of Satan. A human being had to eradicate selfishness with love. It is this renewed human nature, achieved singly by Christ, that God offers to instill in all who trust him. We become partakers of the divine nature, through our trust in Jesus.

SURPRISE FROM HISTORY

Amazingly, this beautiful view of what Christ accomplished, which demonstrates God's incredible character of love, is exactly what was taught by the church fathers in the first two centuries after Christ's resurrection. They called it the doctrine of recapitulation—the idea that Christ came to rebuild or heal humanity in himself.

Justin Martyr (A.D. 103-165) taught that Christ came to do three things: overthrow death, destroy Satan and restore humanity back to God's design, thus providing eternal life to fallen humanity.

(Christ) having been made flesh submitted to be born of the Virgin, in order that through this dispensation the Serpent, who at the first had done evil, and the angels assimilated to him might be put down and death might be despised.[6]

Robert Franks describes Justin's theology as follows:

In fact we find in Justin clear indications of the presence to his mind of the recapitulation theory, afterwards more fully developed by Irenaeus, according to which Christ becomes a new head of humanity, undoes the sin of Adam by reversing the acts and circumstances of his disobedience, and finally communicates to men immortal life.[7]

Franks also describes Irenaeus's (second century A.D., circa 202) theology:

We come here to the famous Irenaean docrtrine of Recapitulation. The conception is that of Christ as the Second Adam, or second head of humanity, who not only undoes the consequences of Adam's fall, but also takes up the development of humanity broken off in him, and carries it to completion, i.e. to union with God and consequent immortality.

"It was God recapitulating the ancient creation of man in himself, that he might slay sin, and annul death, and give life to man." Also III 18, 1: "The Son of God, when he was incarnate and was made man, recapitulated in himself the long line of men, giving us salvation compendiously (*in compendio*), so that what we had lost in Adam, viz. that we should be after in the image and similitude of God, this we should receive in Jesus Christ."[8]

Amazingly, some in the early church understood that Christ's mission was to rebuild humanity back into God's original design. They realized God's law of love was the template on which he built his universe, and they rightly realized that, in order to save humankind, the law on which life is constructed to operate had to be restored into humanity. Christ's mission was to restore humankind back into harmony with God.

The truth of what Christ accomplished, while forgotten by many, continues to be proclaimed by some. In his book *The Nature of the*

Atonement Bruce Reichenbach affirms that sin kills, whereas God, through Christ, heals:

> Why is the death of the Servant or Physician necessary? For most atonement theories this is the heart of the problem. If God is omnipotent and merciful, why demand a route to salvation that exacts the price of the death of God's Son?
>
> Our response can be traced to the virulence of our disease borne by the Servant. What he takes on is no trivial matter; the wages of sin are death (Rom 6:23). Death, in some form, came into the world through sin (Rom 5:12). Christ voluntarily assumes this virulent poison, so strong that it brings death, ours and his, but at the same time not so strong that death can permanently hold the Physician. The death is in the sin. Our sin, not God, kills the Physician. God's part is in mercy to send his Servant/Physician to heal and then to restore him to life and power.[9]

If this is how the early church understood it, if this is what Christ accomplished, then what happened? How have we drifted so far?

GOD'S LAW AND HOW WE HAVE BEEN DECEIVED

A time-tested military strategy is diversion. Create a ruckus in one area, get the enemy focusing on a distraction and then attack from their blind spot.

Magicians, charlatans, and hucksters rely on misdirection as the bedrock of their deceptive craft. They get your attention focused on one action so you don't notice their true intent and, before you know it, you are conned into believing they have power or wisdom—or that they are the best place to invest your money. They know that when you believe you have identified the "trick," figured out the "con," uncovered the "deceit" you will be vulnerable to their real exploit.

Satan, the greatest deceiver in the universe, uses this strategy to near perfection. And God prophesied through Daniel that the evil one would speak against God and seek to change his law (Dan 7:25). For years I, like many other Christians, was bamboozled into believing I knew the devil's lie about God's law, but recently I discovered I had only identified his misdirection.

Some Christians have argued the change in God's law, prophesied by Daniel, occurred when Ten-Commandment law was changed by removing the second commandment, which prohibited making images. Then the tenth commandment was split into two parts (to keep the total number of commandments at ten after deleting the second one), and the sabbath commandment was changed. For more than five hundred years these changes have been a point of contention between various Christian groups.

Diversion—Satan's master misdirection—was what this open change to the Decalogue was. Make an overt, admitted and endorsed change in the law, get everyone focusing on this obvious modification, arguing for or against it, and then infect their minds with the real change they never even notice. Diabolically brilliant.

So what is the real change to God's law, the change Christians almost universally accept as true? *That God's law is an imposed law put on his creatures to govern their lives and test their obedience— rather than the truth that God's law is a natural law, a principle on which he created life to operate.* The devil didn't merely trick Christianity into attempting to change two commandments; he has gotten Christians to accept a change in the very nature of the law itself![10]

Prior to Constantine, Christians recognized God's law as the law of love, the principle on which life is built, and thus they realized Christ's true purpose was to rebuild and restore humanity. But after Constantine converted, the concept of imperialism, with a powerful emperor imposing law on his subjects, gradually infected Christianity. Christians lost sight of God's law of love and instead accepted an imposed law by a powerful potentate. After all, if they still believed God's law was the natural law of love, like the law of respiration, which requires we breathe to live, would they ever have thought a church committee could vote to change such a law?

In his book *Defending Constantine*, Peter Leithart documents that Constantine used the imposition of law to support the church (emphasis mine):

> [Constantine's] rhetoric against both pagans and Jews was forceful, sometimes vicious, and this, along with the *legal restrictions*, created an atmosphere that discouraged but did not destroy paganism. He Christianized public space in Rome, funded the restoration of sacred sites in Palestine and founded Constantinople. . . . When disputes arose in the church, Constantine believed it was his right and duty as Roman emperor to guide the warring factions toward a resolution. . . . Once the bishops had arrived at a decision, Constantine accepted it as a divine word and backed up conciliar decisions with *legal sanctions*, mainly exile for those found guilty of heresy.[11]

Constantine's legal restrictions to support the church not only contributed to the way Christianity viewed God's law but is evidence in itself that God's law was already being viewed as imposed. If Constantine followed the lead of the bishops, then why didn't the bishops refer the emperor to the biblical principle of freedom of conscience (Rom 14:5)? Was it not because they had already lost sight of God's natural law of love and believed God operated just as Constantine was doing? The record of Christianity over the following centuries (the Crusades, the Inquisition) is sad confirmation that the law of love had been replaced with an imposed law-construct.

In this regard, Protestant or Catholic matters not—both have accepted the idea that God's law is imposed and, unavoidably, have accepted the destructive views of God such a belief creates: God as the imperial imposer of law, punisher of lawbreakers, and source of torture and death for all who fail to have their sins paid.

So, bottom line: is God's law imposed, or is it a natural law, a law that was not created, enacted or legislated? Because of God's use of law throughout human history, some may think God's law is both natural and imposed. While God did introduce "laws," these were simply therapeutic interventions to educate and protect until the law of love was put back into the heart. In my book *Could It Be This Simple?* I described this relationship between God's written law and his natural law:

> It [the written law] reveals the defects in our mind. When we recognize those defects, we go to the heavenly Physician for healing. After He has healed us, the written law doesn't need to be destroyed. In fact, when it examines us, it finds no defects because we are in harmony with it. And having been healed, we no longer need the written law. It is the essence of what Paul tells Timothy: "We know that the law is good if one uses it properly. We also know that law is made not for the righteous but for lawbreakers and rebels, the ungodly and sinful, the unholy and irreligious; for those who kill their fathers or mothers, for murderers, for adulterers and perverts, for slave traders and liars and perjurers—and for whatever else is contrary to the sound doctrine that conforms to the glorious gospel of the blessed God, which he entrusted to me" (1 Tim 1.8-11, NIV 1984).

> Using [a] metaphor of an MRI, we might paraphrase the passage like this: "We know that the MRI is good if one uses it properly. We also know that the MRI is made not for healthy people but for those who are sick and diseased, the suffering, the ill, and all those who are dying, and all activities that are contrary to the principles of healthy living that conform to the model of health that the blessed God has entrusted to me."

In fact, the Ten Commandment portion of the law is a special distillation of the great cosmic law of love and liberty written especially for those of us here on this planet. Did the angels in heaven require a law to honor their mother and father? Or to instruct them not to commit adultery? No, but they did need to operate by the law of love and liberty. . . . The

Ten Commandments are a further extrapolation of this law, as Christ himself emphasized: "'Love the Lord your God with all your heart and with all your soul and with all your mind.' This is the first and greatest commandment. And the second is like it: 'Love your neighbor as yourself.' All the Law and the Prophets hang on these two commandments'" (Matt 22:37-40).[12]

It was only after human beings deviated from God's design that the written law became necessary. And its purpose was not to create an imposed governmental system, like Rome, but merely as a diagnostic tool and protective hedge until the day we are fully healed.[13]

It only make sense that when the God who is Love created, he constructed, built and designed everything to operate in harmony with his own nature and character of love, because it is by him that all things hold together (Col 1:17). This is exactly what inspiration reveals: "Love does no harm to a neighbor. Therefore *love is the fulfillment of the law*" (Rom 13:10, emphasis mine).

God's law is the law of love, and this law is the law on which life is designed to operate. Breaking this law automatically results in ruin and death. This reality is clearly described in the book *Hard Sayings of the Bible*: "In some sense, God's wrath is built into the very structure of created reality. In rejecting God's structure and establishing our own, in violating God's intention for the creation and substituting our own intentions, we cause our own disintegration."[14] Death is the inevitable result of breaking the law of love, unless the Designer intervenes to heal and restore (Rom 6:23; Jas 1:15). Christ was sent to do just that, to heal and restore, "For God did not send his Son into the world to condemn the world, but to save the world through him" (Jn 3:17).

SO WHAT IS GOD'S ATONEMENT?

In the mountains of north Georgia is a beautiful Christian youth camp. Established in 1955, it served as a summer retreat for countless

Christian children and families over the years. But in the 1970s a problem arose. Parents started questioning whether to send their children there. Those not associated with the camp began to draw unhealthy conclusions. Attendance was threatened if action wasn't taken. The camp board held meetings to determine what to do. There was only one course they could take to save the camp. They had to change its name, because no Christian parent would send their children to Camp Cumby-Gay.[15]

Words are symbols used to convey ideas and, as society changes, sometimes words can change meanings. If we don't understand the change, we might draw the wrong conclusion.

Atonement is one of those words whose meaning has changed. I remember when I used to believe God's law was an imposed law, it affected how I understood God's Word. Like many, I thought that atonement meant "satisfaction or reparation for a wrong or injury; to make amends." I drew all kinds of wrong conclusions: like Jesus had to die to appease the Father's wrath toward my sin. As long as I be lieved that distortion, love didn't flow in my heart. It was the truth that set me free and opened my heart to love.

I discovered that when the King James Bible was created, being translated into English in 1611, atonement had a different meaning than we typically ascribe today. In the sixteenth and seventeenth centuries the word *one* was not only a noun but also a verb. If two people were at odds and I wanted to bring them back into friendship, I might say, "I am going to *one* them": I am going to bring them back into unity, into oneness. This concept quickly became known as "at-one" or "atone." We pronounce it atone rather than at-one because that is the older English pronunciation. When you are all by yourself, you are not "all one" but "alone." The process of uniting warring factions is, therefore, called atonement.[16]

Jesus is the way back to unity and oneness with God. He came to "at-one" for our sin—to repair the breach sin caused in our relationship with God and reconcile us to himself. Through Jesus, the law of love, the principle of life, is restored within humanity. "This is the covenant I will establish with the people of Israel after that time, declares the Lord. I will put my laws in their minds and write them on their hearts. I will be their God, and they will be my people" (Heb 8:10).

Through the incredibly powerful weapon of perfect love, Jesus crushed the serpent's head (Gen 3:15). In Jesus, love crushed selfishness. "By his [Jesus'] death he might destroy him who holds the power of death—that is, the devil" (Heb 2:14 NIV 1984).

When we as individuals recognize all that Jesus revealed about the Father and finally begin to trust him, we open our hearts and receive, via the work of the Holy Spirit, the transfusion of Christlikeness. The Holy Spirit takes what Christ achieved and reproduces it in us. His victory over evil, his perfect character of righteousness, his nature of love, is "downloaded" into our hearts and we become like him. Our thoughts are brought into harmony with his, our desires in union with his, our character renewed to be like his, our motives cleansed to be like his. We live a Christlike life, for it is no longer I, the sinful, selfish me living, but Christ, the lover of others who lives in me. His perfect love drives out all fear.

Being overwhelmed with the loveliness of God's character, being disgusted with the grossness of our inherent selfishness, falling down in humble submission at the feet of our great, heavenly Physician, and surrendering self to his healing power is called "repentance." It is in our humble repentance, brought about by God's grace, that we experience, via the Holy Spirit, the transfusion of Christ's life and are renewed to a life of love.

Dr. Curt Thompson rightly describes this process beginning here, because of Jesus' victory, and culminating at the second coming of Christ:

> With God's resurrection of Jesus from the dead, Jesus' ascension to his place as Lord of this world, and the outpouring

of the Holy Spirit, God has released the power to integrate our prefrontal cortices. These new neural networks reflect and point to the new heaven and earth that will reach their culmination in the appearance of Jesus but whose shadowy forerunning is already emerging in our lives.[17]

It is in a trust relationship with God, communing and meditating on his love, that our brains—that amazing gathering of gray matter within our skulls—are transformed. The prefrontal cortex grows stronger and its influence extends through the rest of the brain. The limbic system is calmed, distorted ideas are removed, empathy, altruism and giving all increase, and we experience genuine peace and joy.

Only through Jesus is this possible. Only in a trust relationship with him can we ever be healed, because only in Jesus can we know the truth about God, which wins us to trust and, then, in that trust relationship, we experience the transfusion of his character of love. This healing process restores us to his original ideal. Finally, in spite of our humanity, we begin to live by the power of love. At long last, the promise God delivered in Eden will be fulfilled in our own lives: "The God of peace will soon crush Satan under your feet" (Rom 16:20).[18]

Embracing the
Goodness of God

14

Forgiveness

We must develop and maintain the capacity to forgive.
He who is devoid of the power to forgive
is devoid of the power to love.

MARTIN LUTHER KING JR.

MARIA WAS NOT MY PATIENT but a member of my church. As she approached me one day after services, I could see the anguish in her eyes. She was obviously struggling with something; I could tell she was in turmoil. She spoke with a heavy accent and her words were hesitant, uncertain. She was obviously afraid, and I couldn't tell what frightened her most—that I might not answer her question or that the answer I would give would cause her deeper concern.

She told me that her only daughter, Sylvia, was twenty-five years old and had recently married a young man named Hector. She had concerns about Hector prior to the marriage but never voiced them, deciding that if this was the man her daughter was going to marry she would do all she could to support them. The wedding was eight months ago and, under the circumstances as she came to know them, Maria could no longer be supportive.

It was only two weeks after they returned from the honeymoon that Hector first hit Sylvia. Initially Sylvia covered the bruises and kept the pain to herself. She made excuses in her mind: *He didn't mean it. He was tired. I upset him. I know he loves me.* But as the weeks passed and the beatings became more frequent and severe, the young bride could no longer keep the truth hidden and, a couple of months ago, her mother found out. Since then, Sylvia had been coming over to the house on an almost weekly basis tattooed with new injuries.

Understandably, Maria was enraged. She confronted Hector, who responded with a detached indifference, looking at Maria with a sadistic pleasure in his eyes. The more she pled for her daughter and the greater her distress over Sylvia's mistreatment, the more Hector seemed to enjoy it. She hated him, despised him, and the rage inside her was building to volcanic force.

Maria had lost her peace. She thought constantly of her daughter and Hector's abuse. She counseled her daughter to leave her husband, but Sylvia reminded her of the sanctity of marriage and her commitment to stay. Sylvia continued to make excuses for Hector and to submit to his endless abuse. Maria's anger built. She tossed and turned at night, unable to get the battered images of Sylvia from her mind—or purge her dreams of the battering she'd like to deliver to her son-in-law.

Sin is insidious. We barely notice when it begins to grow in our hearts. Like a deadly virus infecting first one person, then another, we pass sin to others without a care—infecting them with a cutting comment, cruel laugh, retaliatory strike or cold shoulder. Every injury cherished, every slight retained, every wound unhealed remains a festering pocket of evil's seed, germinating more injury, spreading more pain and suffering. Maria's heart was infected and she barely knew it.

Church, the one place Maria had always found comfort and peace, had become empty to her. She heard the stories of God's love, of Jesus' sacrifice, but her heart burned with bitterness, resentment and rage. She wanted "justice." She wanted God to rain fire down from heaven and destroy Hector. She wanted to see him pay. She knew the Bible said to forgive, but she didn't want forgiveness. She wanted vengeance.

Maria's limbic system was inflamed, and her prefrontal cortex was being impaired. Love was not flowing in her mind. Instead she ruminated on vengeful themes, which further fueled her anger. She acknowledged the hatred, anger and bitterness in her heart, and embraced it as a desire for "justice." Sin's evil virus infecting her heart was taking hold and, if not cut out, would destroy her.

Maria's problem was not Hector. Maria's problem was the anger, hatred and rage burning in her heart toward Hector. If she wanted peace, she had to excise this poisonous unforgiveness from her heart. I told Maria that God has given us only one weapon to free our hearts from such turmoil: forgiveness. If she wanted peace, she must forgive Hector.

But that's not what Maria wanted to hear. She wanted a solution that would gratify her desire for revenge, a solution that would cause Hector pain. She wanted a god who would condone her desire for retributions. She became angry with me then, and she turned and walked away.

Such a desire for vengeance is the reason so many people cling to lies about God. In such cases, we actually *want* a god who is vengeful and severe, who will gratify our selfish desire for retribution. The truth about our heavenly Father would heal the prefrontal cortex, which would result in calming the limbic system and relinquishing the demand for vengeance. Only by holding to lies about God can the brain continue to pursue the hateful course.

Sin is sneaky. Hector had not directly sinned against Maria; Hector's sin was against Sylvia. But his abuse of Sylvia instilled a cruel desire in Maria's heart, a malignancy that was already starting to bear the pernicious tumor of hatred, spite and rage that, if not removed, would eventually take over all goodness in Maria's heart. If radical, spiritual heart surgery was not performed soon, Maria would become as hard-hearted as Hector.

FORGIVENESS: THE VACCINE FOR SIN

It is by forgiving those who mistreat, abuse and exploit us that we obstruct the spread of sin. Through forgiveness, we halt the plague of selfishness. Through forgiveness, we destroy the toxin of bitterness, resentment and desire for retaliation. Through forgiveness, we not only inoculate ourselves, we spread the antidote to sin—the love of God.

It is our privilege to receive God's love and forgiveness, and to let that love flow through us to the world. By forgiving others, we disseminate the only antidote to evil and sin. But love doesn't flow where lies are retained. Sadly, far too many people have accepted a false antidote, the worthless potion peddled by that old serpent, the original snake-oil salesman—the devil. Many, instead of freely forgiving, have advanced (under the guise of godliness), a policy of "stern justice" and "righteous retribution"—the elixir of Satan.

God is working through Jesus to bring the universe back into unity with himself (Jn 17:20-21; Eph 1:10). But the doctrine of "justice," rather than reconciling this world to God and unifying people in love to each other, inflames hostilities, increases hatred and causes divisions to grow ever deeper. Surely this is the venom of the serpent.

BIBLICAL JUSTICE

On September 20, 2011, just nine days after terrorists attacked the United States in four hijacked passenger jets, President George W. Bush addressed a joint session of Congress. In that speech, President Bush stated, "Whether we bring our enemies to justice or bring justice to our enemies, justice will be done."[1]

His point was clear: the United States would hunt down and inflict punishment on those responsible for that heinous crime. Do you think the president's words reflected God's attitude toward wayward humanity? Does the "justice" of a vengeful nation accurately represent the justice of God?

Is it right to conclude God runs his universe like sinful beings run earthly governments? Or do we misrepresent God and obstruct his healing love when we construe God's justice to be like our own?

Was Jesus suggesting God's government is different from ours when he said, "My kingdom is not of this world" (Jn 18:36)? Is there a reason the Bible uses ferocious beasts to represent earthly governments but a lamb to represent Jesus? Could this suggest something different about how the two systems operate? Could human justice and God's justice be different?

Is God, in Isaiah 55, revealing his methods to be drastically different than fallen humanity?

> Let the wicked forsake his way
>   and the evil man his thoughts.
> Let him turn to the LORD, and he will have mercy on him,
>   and to our God, for he will *freely pardon*.
>
> *"For my thoughts are not your thoughts,*
>   *Neither are your ways my ways,"*
>   declares the LORD.
> "As the heavens are higher than the earth,
>   so are *my ways higher than your ways*
>   *and my thoughts higher than your thoughts.*
> As the rain and the snow
>   come down from heaven,
> and do not return to it
>   without watering the earth
> and making it bud and flourish,
>   so that it yields seed for the sower and bread for the eater,
>   so is my word that goes out from my mouth." (Is 55:7-11
>   NIV 1984, emphasis mine)

In describing how he freely pardons and how his law of love operates to bring life to the earth, was God stating that his government, his way of doing things, is not like ours? Could his justice be different than what sinful beings practice?

Justice in any system is based on the law of that organization. Punching someone in the face is just in boxing but unjust in baseball. The rules of the various sports governing bodies determine what a just or unjust action is. Driving at 160 miles per hour on the autobahn in Germany is just (or right), but not so in the United States because the United States has a different set of laws. Justice in God's government is built on God's law, and God's law is the law of love. Therefore, God's justice is always an expression of God's character of love:

> Defend the poor and the fatherless; uphold the cause of the poor and the oppressed. (Ps 82:3)

> Wash yourselves clean. Stop all this evil that I see you doing. Yes, stop doing evil and learn to do right. See that justice is done—help those who are oppressed, give orphans their rights, and defend widows. (Is 1:16-17 GNT)

> The LORD longs to be gracious to you; he rises to show you compassion. The LORD is a God of justice. (Is 30:18 NIV 1984)

> This is what the LORD says to the dynasty of David: 'Give justice each morning to the people you judge! Help those who have been robbed; rescue them from their oppressors.' (Jer 21:12 NLT)

The amazing truth that we have somehow forgotten is that biblical justice is *delivering the oppressed, not punishing the oppressor!*

Justice presented as infliction of punishment in order to avenge is a human concept, and it infects our theology when we accept imposed law-concepts. But the imposition of discipline to teach, heal and restore is an expression of love and is consistent with God's methods and principles.

When we remember God's law is the protocol on which life is built, then we remember that violations of God's law are incompatible with eternal life, that we are born in a terminal condition and, therefore, the infliction of punishment is not needed. However, loving discipline to save, before eternal ruin occurs, *is* often needed. One never has to inflict punishment on those who violate the laws of health; the violation brings its own punishment. But many an adolescent has benefited from the loving discipline of parents when caught with a cigarette or beer. What the justice of love requires is healing, rescue, restoration. The question is, through which law do you view justice?

After presenting these concepts during a weekly Bible study class, I received the following email from an online listener:

> Previously I attended your class for two weeks back in 2009. You might remember that I was previously a [Christian] pastor for fifteen years. I am currently enrolled in law school. . . .
>
> I was receiving this week's outline where you stated: "When one accepts that God imposes law, then one must conclude that the consequences one experiences for disobedience to God's law is imposed by God, or that God's wrath is something that he inflicts to punish for sin."
>
> Since I am [in law school, I am] developing my views of criminal punishment and civil sanctions. Should I relate my view of God into the courtroom? More specifically, there are two views of punishment, utilitarianism and retributivism.
>
> Utilitarianism seeks to reform the criminal, reason with the criminal, and the focus is on therapy and psychiatric care. This view also incarcerates the criminal to convince the general community to forgo criminal conduct in the future. Finally it teaches the convicted what conduct is impermissible.
>
> Retributivism seeks to punish the criminal for freely violating the rules. This view gratifies the passion for revenge. Retributive punishment is the means of securing a moral balance in society where the inmate pays back his debt to society. Retributivism seeks punishment as a way to right a wrong and corrects the claim.

It appears that the wrong view of God has much in common with the retributivism view of criminal punishment. While the utilitarianism view of criminal punishment has much in common with the restoration view of salvation.

But should I look to the heart-wise, healing, loving picture of God view when it comes to criminals? Should my decision of how I view God relate to what punishment a murderer, rapist, burglar, and thief receives? In other words, should I be using my influence to end punishment of criminals? So criminals can be set free from prison and be placed in rehabilitation groups, therapy, etc. Or suppose criminals were not sent to jail, just allow them to reap the natural consequence of their sins?

His concerns are quite legitimate and are expressed by many as they consider God's law of love. Many people get confused about God's law because God, just like a loving parent, has used imposed rules as stopgaps to help his immature people.

When a mother puts a rule in place not to play in the street lest the child get spanked, the real problem in breaking the rule is not the spanking (imposed penalty) but the violation of the natural law of physics when a car collides with the body of a child. The imposed rule, with its imposed penalty, is intended to protect the child, the unknown driver and even the parent from the result of violation of natural law if the child is hit by a car. The spanking is not intended as retribution but is a stopgap to help keep the child safe until the child is mature enough to govern itself and not play in the street.

In our Christian lives, understanding God's design but operating in a world of sin, a world filled with immature beings who don't understand God's principle for life, we often need to use imposed laws/rules to help protect the innocent from the immature and to protect the immature from themselves. But we should not confuse such imposed interventions with God's ideal for life. We must remember the real purpose for the stopgaps of imposed laws.

The immature need to learn that behavior has consequences. In other words, for every action there is a reaction. The universe operates on natural law, and our choices bring results; healthy choices bring healthy results, and unhealthy choices bring unhealthy results. Imposed human laws are a means to teach this principle, as well as to protect the innocent from those too immature to practice healthy principles, and even to protect the offenders from themselves.

Retribution is a concept of the sinful human mind. It does no good to those offended; it doesn't resurrect the murdered person; it doesn't heal the broken bone; it doesn't restore one's innocence nor does it recover stolen goods. It also doesn't help heal, develop, save or transform the sinner/criminal.

Utilitarianism, which I like to think of as rehabilitation, is focused on protecting *both* society from the criminal and the criminal from damaging himself by continued actions in violation of God's design for life. Each act of selfishness actually damages the sinner, searing the conscience, warping the character, hardening the heart. Putting someone in prison, where they can cease their destructive behavior, can provide an opportunity for reflection, reevaluation and rehabilitation, while also protecting the innocent. But allowing one to continue on destructive rampages not only harms society but ensures the eventual eternal destruction of the criminal.

So in a world of sin, governments act in redemptive ways by intervening in the lives of those who, when they commit crimes, are violating the principles of love. Arrest, prosecution and appropriate punishments are stand-in consequences—like spanking for playing in the road—intended to teach the person that such behaviors are damaging and destructive, while simultaneously protecting society. Incarceration may result in rehabilitation for some, but there are others who have persisted in destructive living so long that they have permanently destroyed the faculties that respond to love and truth—and thus are beyond rehabilitation. For them, incarceration becomes the earthly means of limiting the extent of individual destructive behavior.

A loving person seeks the most effective means of making society a truly safe place. And what would be the safest society? One filled with many prisons, guards and police at every corner? Or a society filled with people who love others more than themselves and would rather die than hurt another? While incarceration is sadly a necessity in the world in which we live, to the degree we can rehabilitate people so that they actually become mature individuals who respect the rights of others, we have done more good for society than retribution ever can.

Let us incarcerate with hearts that love the criminal, that want to see the person redeemed, saved, restored, or if that is not possible, then to see them safe from doing more harm. Jesus commends his followers for not only feeding the hungry but for visiting those in prison (Mt 25:36). Wasn't Jesus encouraging us to seek to redeem, rehabilitate and bring salvation to the criminal? This is God's justice, doing what is right by healing, transforming and saving his children.

God does what is right or just when he takes those out of harmony with his design for life and sets them right, when he renews their hearts, when he turns enemies into friends:

> Anyone who is joined to Christ is a new being; the old is gone, the new has come. All this is done by God, who through Christ *changed us from enemies into his friends and gave us the task of making others his friends also. Our message is that God was making the whole human race his friends* through Christ. God did not keep an account of their sins, and he has given us the message which tells how he makes them his friends.
>
> Here we are, then, speaking for Christ, as though God himself were making his appeal through us. We plead on Christ's behalf: *let God change you from enemies into his friends!* (2 Cor 5:17-20 GNT)

God's law is the natural law on which life is built to operate. Breaking this law automatically results in death, unless the Designer intervenes to heal and restore—to change us from his enemies to his friends. Thus we find God, working through Christ, not punishing sinners but *delivering* those oppressed by sin!

As Jesus said, he came to deliver us:

> The Spirit of the Lord is on me, because he has anointed me to proclaim good news to the poor. He has sent me to proclaim freedom for the prisoners and recovery of sight for the blind, to set the oppressed free, to proclaim the year of the Lord's favor. (Lk 4:18-19)

And Matthew describes Jesus' activities of healing the sick and setting free the demon-possessed to be the fulfillment of God's justice:

> Aware of this, Jesus withdrew from that place. Many followed him, and he *healed all their sick*, warning them not to tell who he was. *This was to fulfill what was spoken through the prophet Isaiah:*
>
> "Here is my servant whom I have chosen,
>   the one I love, in whom I delight;
> I will put my Spirit on him,
>   and *he will proclaim justice to the nations.*
> He will not quarrel or cry out;
>   no one will hear his voice in the streets.
> A bruised reed he will not break,
>   and a smoldering wick he will not snuff out,
> *till he leads justice to victory.*
>   In his name the nations will put their hope."
>
> Then they brought him a demon-possessed man who was blind and mute, and Jesus *healed him*, so that he could both talk and see. (Mt 12:15-22 NIV 1984, emphasis mine)

But there are dangerous societal consequences to believing God is forgiving while continuing to hold the idea that God's law is imposed. A 2012 study conducted by the department of psychology at the University of Oregon, after accounting for multiple covariants, found that belief in a punishing God reduces crime, whereas belief in a benevolent God predicts higher crime.[2]

Why would belief in a punishing God reduce crime, whereas belief in a benevolent God result in higher crime? The problem is not accepting the truth that God is merciful, but it is believing the lie that God's law is like a Roman emperor's and that God's government operates like human governments. I am confident that if a municipality posted speed limits, but also broadcast that 100 percent of those caught speeding would always be pardoned, speeding would increase. When we have an imposed law, failure to impose penalties results in worsening crime.

When we accept imperial Rome's imposed law-concept as God's law, we distort the divine character and teach that, when the law gets broken, God must use his power to inflict punishment on lawbreakers. God's justice is no longer seen as deliving the oppressed, but like post-9/11 America, hunting down and destroying the oppressors. Therefore, if God isn't hunting us down to torture and kill, we falsely believe there is no punishment for sin and crime rises.

But what if everyone realized life can only exist in harmony with God's law of love? What if people remembered that those who commit crimes against others, while they can hurt another's body, cannot warp another's character? What if people knew that when one commits a crime against another they are actually searing their own consciences, warping their own characters, destroying their own souls—the natural result of operating outside God's design for life?

Jesus said, "Do not be afraid of those who kill the body but cannot kill the soul" (Mt 10:28). The Greek word for soul is ψυχή, *psychē*, from which we get *psyche* and *psychology* and *psychiatry*. It means our unique individuality, personhood or identity. Evil people can sin against us, even destroy our bodies, but another person cannot sully our souls. But when we commit evil against another we harden our hearts and take ourselves further out of harmony with God's design for life. The problem is not in believing God is merciful but in misunderstanding God's law. It all comes back to how you understand God's character and law.

AN EYE FOR AN EYE

Bob's anger was evident: he was seething. His face glowed red and the veins were bulging on his forehead. Six months earlier, while his sister was at his house, Bob had had too much to drink and had fallen asleep. While he was sleeping, his sister stole the rare coin collection Bob had started in childhood. She took the coins, left the state and sold them to get money to buy drugs. Bob was furious.

For the following six months he was irritable, flying off the handle at the most minor inconvenience and accusing friends of slights that had never occurred. He was alienating people at work and home. He had come to see me at the insistence of his wife, who reported that he'd become a monster to live with and, if he didn't get help, she was moving out.

Bob refused to forgive his sister. He wanted to make her pay. He wanted to hold her accountable. He wanted to wring her neck! Bob wanted "justice" and wouldn't forgive until he got it.

The truth was that Bob had accepted the lie, the false remedy to sin, the distortion about God. As his limbic system strengthened and his prefrontal cortex weakened, his ability to be kind, understanding, compassionate, patient and gentle diminished. He took his faltering brain with him wherever he went, and all of his relationships began to suffer. He could not get well until he accepted and applied the truth, because love cannot flow where lies are retained.

Sadly, many of us are so steeped in lies about God that we fail to see his loving hand. Believing God to be a being of stern justice, who must inflict penalties in order to be just and who must be appeased in order to be kind, we fail to recognize therapeutic discipline done in love. Instead, like Bob, we too often see loving discipline as acts of vengeance:

If anyone takes the life of a human being, he must be put to death. Anyone who takes the life of someone's animal must make restitution—life for life. If anyone injures his neighbor, whatever he has done must be done to him: fracture for fracture, eye for eye, tooth for tooth. As he has injured the other, so he is to be injured. (Lev 24:17-20 NIV 1984)

I remember a time when I thought like Bob. I wanted others to pay for any wrong they had done to me. In those days, I also used the above passage to justify cruelty, claiming virtue in the process. But Gandhi was right: "An eye for an eye leaves the whole world blind."[3] It was only when I looked through the eyes of Jesus that I saw something different. I wondered, *What if God gave these instructions to a group of people who killed an offender for any misdeed—imparting death for the most insignificant misdemeanor? What if he gave these instructions to a group of people who would eventually kill their King, who was blameless?* In that situation, would God be severe or would he be graciously taking a brutish people and moving them toward mercy, toward grace and toward forgiveness? After careful, prayerful study, I realized that was exactly what God was doing. Sadly, even today, God still struggles to free our minds from such distortions about him.

A SHEPHERD BOY

On August 7, 2006, journalist John Hendren filed a report for National Public Radio from the Iraqi war zone. Mr. Hendren investigated the cause of the high number of civilian casualties that were occurring in that war-torn country. He described one shepherd boy, no older than twelve, who while playing, threw a stone that accidently hit a man's cow, blinding one of that animal's eyes. The farmer shot and killed the boy. God's instruction in Leviticus was for people like that farmer: people too hard-hearted to conceive of outright forgiveness; people too self-centered to pardon; people too selfish to love others as God loves us.

Fifteen hundred years later, Jesus confirms the true meaning of the Leviticus 24 passage. It is only by loving others that evil is vanquished, only by forgiving others that God's kingdom is advanced:

You have heard that it was said, "Eye for eye, and tooth for tooth." But I tell you, Do not resist an evil person. If someone strikes you on the right cheek, turn to him the other also. And if someone wants to sue you and take your tunic, let him have your cloak as well. If someone forces you to go one mile, go with him two miles. Give to the one who asks you, and do not turn away from the one who wants to borrow from you.

You have heard that it was said, "Love your neighbor and hate your enemy." But I tell you: Love your enemies and pray for those who persecute you, that you may be sons of your Father in heaven. (Mt 5:38-45 NIV 1984)

When we forgive others, we not only halt the expansion of sin but we free ourselves from its power and grip. By forgiving others we strengthen the prefrontal cortex, calm the limbic system and become conduits of God's healing love.

I DON'T LIKE YOU VERY MUCH

I met Robert during a business trip to West Palm Beach, Florida, in March 2008. I was there presenting a series of lectures on neurobiology, and for two days he drove me to and from the speaking venues.

Robert was an intelligent man who talked openly about his faith in God and love for him. During our time together I talked about God's unconditional love and the power of forgiveness, and of giving oneself for another. After thoughtful contemplation one day he said, "I don't know. If some crackhead broke into my house and was threatening my wife and daughter, and I had a gun, I would shoot him."

"Okay," I replied, "Imagine a twenty-year-old crackhead, crazed out of his mind, breaks into your house. He is confused and obviously psychotic from the drugs, and is threatening your family. And yes, you have a gun. But the crackhead just happens to be your firstborn son. Now what would you do?"

Robert glanced over at me with a frown and said, "I don't like you very much."

This imaginary scenario represents God's position. We are all his beloved, and he is trying to save every one of us. He is trying to bring each of us back into unity with him, back to where we love others more than ourselves. It is when we love others more than ourselves, when we freely forgive, that the spread of evil is obstructed.

A SOLDIER OF LOVE

During World War II, sixteen million men served in the U.S. armed forces, and of that number, only 431 displayed such heroism as to be awarded the Congressional Medal of Honor. I had the privilege of knowing one of those men. His complete story can be found in the book *The Unlikeliest Hero*.

Desmond Doss was a devout Christian from the southern Appalachian Mountains who willingly entered the military when his draft number came up in 1942. Because of his religious beliefs, he had obtained the written permission of the President of the United States and the Army Chief of Staff not to bear arms, to serve as a conscientious objector.

Doss actually protested the term "conscientious objector," preferring the term "conscientious *cooperator*." He said he was glad to serve his country; he just could not take another life. But that didn't go over too well in the 1940s.

Life in the army was not easy, and it was especially tough for those who refused to bear arms. During training with the 77th Infantry Division, private Doss was mocked, ridiculed, scorned and mistreated. When he refused to accept a rifle for training, he was pressured, criticized, pled with and threatened. Some members of his unit were so disgruntled that they threatened to kill him when they got into combat. In the barracks, boots and other objects were often thrown at him in the night. But Doss took solace in God and his daily Bible study and prayer.

Doss consistently requested to be moved from the infantry company to a medical battalion and finally, with the intervention of the unit chaplain, he was assigned to medics training and moved to the combat support battalion of the 77th. Along with other medics, he learned how to bandage wounds, stop bleeding, apply tourniquets and administer other first aid. But the ridicule, harassment and resentment from members of his unit continued.

Eventually, his unit was deployed to the Pacific Theater and saw one bloody conflict after another: Guam, Leyte and Okinawa. Army intelligence reports confirmed that Japanese soldiers were instructed to hunt for and kill medics first as a way to demoralize the troops. Doss's commander ordered him to carry a rifle as a way to disguise the fact that he was a medic, but Doss refused. His battalion commander attempted to have him sent back to the States before their first action, but Doss's company commander interceded and he stayed with his unit.

Despite all the harassment, Doss maintained a forgiving attitude toward his comrades. Between 1944 and 1945 Doss selflessly exposed himself to enemy fire repeatedly to save members of his unit, many of whom had mistreated him. His persistently gracious and selfless actions eventually won the admiration of his entire division. In one battle alone Doss was credited by his commander with single-handedly saving a hundred men, lowering them down a 400-foot escarpment—while continuously exposed to enemy fire. Despite a head count confirming the number, Doss protested, believing it just couldn't have been that many, so the commander agreed to lower the number in the official citation to seventy-five. The commendation concludes with these words:

Through his outstanding bravery and unflinching determination in the face of desperately dangerous conditions Pfc. Doss saved the lives of many soldiers. His name became a symbol throughout the 77th Infantry Division for outstanding gallantry far above and beyond the call of duty.

Desmond Doss never held a grudge but maintained a forgiving heart through those many months of training. It is by forgiving those who injure us that we free ourselves and become agents to minister God's love. If Doss had "kept score," counted up misdeeds, kept record of wrongs against him, his heart would have been filled with fear, and he could never have been used so powerfully by the God he worshiped. It was by forgiving others that his heart remained open to be a conduit of God's healing love.

APPLICATION

Practice examining the three threads of evidence. Do you find harmonious evidence in Scripture, in God's testable laws and in experience for the healing principle of forgiveness? Does the evidence provided by the life of Christ confirm that forgiveness is part of God's character and methods? How did Christ treat those who crucified him?

Examine your own experience and identify times in which you have wronged another and experienced forgiveness, and when someone refused to forgive you but instead held resentment and bitterness toward you. What impact did each experience have on you and them?

Then examine times in your life when you have been offended and you forgave easily and quickly, versus times in which you held resentment over an offense before forgiving—or perhaps you're still holding onto resentment. Was the experience different to forgive freely than to hold resentment? What was different? In which experience did you find healing and peace more quickly? What happened to the relationship in which you forgave versus the one in which you held resentment?[4]

15

When Good Prevails

Love many things, for therein lies the true strength,
and whosoever loves much performs much,
and can accomplish much, and what
is done in love is done well.

VINCENT VAN GOGH

WE HAVE EXPLORED VARIOUS VIEWS OF GOD and discovered that perspectives that increase love are healing, while those that incite fear are destructive. In this chapter we will explore this application in actual scenarios of other-centered love to see how love overcomes our natural fear instincts.

LOVE AND WEDDING DAY FEARS

Barbara came to see me on her own. She had a lifelong history of fear, anxiety and worry. While she worried about bills, her children and her family's health, her primary fear centered on what others thought of her. She didn't like herself, feared rejection and, therefore, was terrified of activities in which she would be the center of attention. She was afraid of speaking in public and declined almost all invitations for parties or social gatherings. If she did find herself in a group event, she would gravitate to a corner and try to blend in with the wallpaper.

But catastrophe loomed just weeks away. Barbara's daughter was getting married. For the last three months, as the wedding date approached, Barbara's anxiety had been steadily rising. With each passing day the pressure and tension built until she was nearing collapse. In desperation she came to see me. Why was Barbara dreading the event? Not because of any concerns about the match her daughter had made. Barbara was terrified because mothers are seated last at weddings: she would have to walk down the aisle with everyone looking at her. Her anxiety had become so excruciating she was actually thinking of not going to her own daughter's wedding.

As soon as I discovered the source of her anxiety, I realized what she needed. She needed the law of love. She needed to get the focus off herself and onto another. So I said, "Whose special day will that be?"

"My daughter's."

"And who are you focusing on?"

She hung her head and said, "Myself."

I challenged her, "Why not try taking the focus off yourself? Think about your daughter, her happiness, how much it will mean to her to have Mom sitting right down there in front. Think about the joy your daughter will experience that day. Think of how you can give of yourself to bless her." I knew that love overcomes fear, that her anterior cingulate cortex (part of her prefrontal cortex where we experience love, empathy and altruism) needed to be activated with love for her daughter. If she could do this, her limbic system would calm and her experience would change.

She came back to see me after the wedding. "I can't believe it," she said with a smile. "I wasn't nervous or anxious at all. I just kept thinking about my daughter, how beautiful she looked in her wedding dress, how happy she was. I thought how glad she would be for me to be there and I just walked right down that aisle without any fear at all."

"Perfect love drives out fear" (1 Jn 4:18). Love heals! Love eradicates fear. The only power in the universe that can heal our hearts and free us from fear is the power of love.

Imagine stepping out into the street and, as you do, you see an eighteen-wheeler bearing down on you. What emotion do you experience? Fear! Imagine your three-year-old son toddles out into that same street. Now the eighteen-wheeler is bearing down on him. There is just enough time to run and push your child out of the way, but if you do, you will get hit. What do you do? You push your child out of the way! And as you see your child roll to safety in the grass, what emotion do you experience? Joy! In both situations you are being hit by a truck; in the first, there is only fear, but in the second, love has vanquished fear.

Love is the only power that can heal us and free us from fear. It cannot be commanded. It cannot be coerced. It cannot be forced. It can only be freely given. Our fear-ridden hearts cannot produce this love; we can only receive this love from God and let it flow through us to others.

LOVE VERSUS LUST

Charlie came to see me despondent, discouraged and hopeless. I was his last stop before he was to carry out his plan to kill himself. He said he came to see me at his wife's insistence, not because he believed I could actually help him but because, at this point in his life, he didn't think it could hurt.

He told me he had never felt good about himself. Often he was the butt of jokes, teased and harassed. He hated school, where he was not part of any group and had very few friends. He sat alone during lunch and never went on a date. He was lonely, hurt and afraid. He feared rejection, feared being laughed at, feared what others thought of him. It was in high school that he first got involved with pornography. When he felt rejected, when he felt lonely, when he felt worthless, he turned to porn. Rather than grappling with his own powerful emotions, rather than working through the hurt, he ran inward, isolating himself from reality. He created a fantasy world revolving around pornographic images.

After graduating high school Charlie's social life improved. College was much less stressful, peers didn't seem to judge or mock him, and soon he had some friends. But porn remained his release. When things got stressful, when emotions got intense, when he began to worry about rejection or what others thought, he immersed himself in his habit. And as he did, his situation only worsened. He lost respect for himself. His conscience convicted him. He was ashamed, guilt-ridden and unsure of himself. Yet he didn't know what to do. He wanted to change but was overwhelmed by the powerful feelings that paralyzed him.

So Charlie kept doing what he knew how to do: he ran. He ran from himself and from his fears, insecurities, guilt, inadequacy and shame, and he sought solace in the arms of women—this time real ones. Charlie knew many women, but no matter how many he got involved with, he still felt empty, lonely and worthless. Even after he married, his condition only worsened. Whenever he and his wife would disagree, argue or experience stress, Charlie would run from himself, his emotions and his responsibilities back to his pornographic fantasies.

Charlie lived in fear—fear of rejection, fear of failure, fear of never overcoming. He had given up hope that he could change. He had given up on himself. He was one step short of permanently running away when he came to see me. Charlie needed love—not the cheap counterfeit in which he had immersed himself but the love that gives for another.

Over the course of treatment, I let Charlie know that I cared for him and slowly built a therapeutic alliance—a relationship in which Charlie felt safe. It was a battle for him. He took many steps to avoid temptation, like not having a computer or Internet access, avoiding basically all TV, where readily available sexual images incited cravings for porn. While such interventions were necessary and helpful, they alone would not heal his heart.

Charlie needed not only to be loved but to love others, to care about others more than self. His prefrontal cortex needed to activate with empathy and compassion for others in order to overcome his limbic-system urges for self-gratification. So during one session I asked him to imagine visiting a porn website and clicking through the pictures—one naked girl after another—until the next one to pop up was a picture of his nineteen-year-old daughter.

His reaction was immediate and powerful. With a look of disgust he said, "That would be awful!"

"You wouldn't enjoy it?"

"Of course not! I can hardly stand to think about it." His voice started to sound irritated.

Looking straight at him, I said, "Every one of those girls is some-body's daughter."

He sat stunned. He didn't say anything for quite some time. Finally, he admitted that the people in those images were never people to him, but objects. Thinking about those girls being his daughter—or someone else's pride and joy—removed all pleasure from that vile habit. Charlie was starting to love. As he came to actually think about the women on those sites—about their dignity, health, welfare—as he allowed himself to care for them, like a father, he no longer found pleasure in porn. His addiction was broken. Love had set him free. Love was now present in his life, busy trampling the serpent under his feet.

SHOOT ME FIRST

October 2, 2006, started out like so many other days in Lancaster County, Pennsylvania: up early, complete morning chores, a hearty breakfast and then off to school. Thirteen-year-old Marian Fisher and her eleven-year-old sister, Barbie, had no idea what would tran-spire that day. So off they went, to their one-room school house in the village of Nickel Mines, Pennsylvania.

At 10:25 a.m., Charles Carl Roberts IV, a thirty-two-year-old milk-truck driver, entered the school carrying a 9-millimeter pistol. He then ordered the boys he found to carry lumber, a shotgun, a stun gun, wires, chains, nails, tools and other items into the school. Next, he sent out fifteen boys, a pregnant woman and two women with infants, then nailed two-by-fours and two-by-sixes across the entrance.

He used strips of plastic and lengths of wire to tie the ankles and wrists of the ten remaining elementary-school students, all girls. It is unclear what his true intentions were, but when the police arrived, he became angry, desperate and increasingly agitated. At 11:07 a.m., when it became obvious he was intent on killing the girls, love stepped in.

Thirteen-year-old Marian Fisher stood up and asked to be shot first. Offering her life in the hope her sister and friends would be set free, she was heard by the survivors to say, "Shoot me and leave the other ones loose."[1] The gunman shot and killed Marian. No sooner had her lifeless body crumpled to the floor than her eleven-year-old sister, Barbie, stood up and said, "Shoot me next," also hoping to save the other girls. The gunman then shot Barbie. She was wounded in the hand, leg and shoulder, but survived.

Charles Roberts killed five of the girls and critically wounded the other five before turning the gun on himself, ending his own life. But it's the incredible selflessness of Marian and Barbie that will be remembered for generations to come. Again we see self-forsaking love at work (Jn 15:13).

Love is not afraid. Love does not seek to protect itself. Love is outrageous. It gives all for others.

Every day the battle rages—love others or seek self. There are only two options in life, two paths, two destinations, two principles, two choices and, ultimately, two kinds of people. The Bible calls them the "wheat and tares," "sheep and goats," "fruitful and withered vine," "pure woman and harlot," "righteous and wicked," "saved and lost." But at its root, love comes down to focusing more on others than self, giving rather than taking. In every act of life, these two principles—love others or seek self—fight for control of our hearts.

WHEN CHRIST IS IN THE HEART

October 4, 2006, Lancaster County, Pennsylvania—two days after the deadly shooting of the ten Amish girls, the Amish community demonstrated love in action, forgiveness without reservation, when they gathered to raise money for the killer's family.

The *World Net Daily* reported,

In what's being called a stunning example of "the imitation of Christ," the Amish community, devastated by the cold-blooded murder of five of its schoolgirls, is raising money for the killer's family. Amish residents of rural Lancaster County, Pa., have started a charity fund to help not only the victims' families — but also the mass-murderer's widow and children. . . .

Dwight Lefever, a spokesman for the Roberts family, said an Amish neighbor comforted the killer's family and extended forgiveness to them after the shooting. And columnist Rod Dreher, reacting to the Amish outpouring of support for the killer's family, wrote: "Yesterday on *NBC News*, I saw an Amish midwife who had helped birth several of the girls murdered by the killer say that they were planning to take food over to his family's house. She said—and I paraphrase closely—'This is possible if you have Christ in your heart.'[2]

LOVE RISKS ALL

August 18, 2001, Orlando, Florida—fifteen-year-old Edna Wilks, her friend Amanda Valance and several other friends had just finished their first week as high-school freshmen. To celebrate, they met together at Lake Conway for a late-night swim. It was a warm night. The sky was clear, and everyone was upbeat.

Shortly after entering the water, Edna felt something brush her left arm. At first she thought it was just one of her friends, but then she saw an alligator surface next to her. Before she could scream, it grabbed her and pulled her under. Later she said, "It started spinning me over and over, and I heard something crack in my body. I'm thinking, *I'm going to die like this.*"

But then, for an instant, the gator loosed its grip and Edna burst to the surface, screaming for help. But everyone else was swimming to shore as fast as they could. Edna began screaming, "Come back! Don't leave me! Please don't leave me!" But everyone did leave; everyone, that is, except her best friend Amanda.

Amanda said, "I thought, *No I can't leave my best friend out there to die.*" So Amanda grabbed her boogie board and swam as fast as she could to where Edna was floating in the water. When she reached her, Edna was bleeding badly. Just then the gator surfaced a few feet away and started moving toward them. Amanda didn't hesitate. She quickly slid off her board, pushed Edna onto it and began swimming as hard as she could for the shore fifty yards away. The gator swam in their direction and suddenly submerged, disappearing from sight. Amanda was terrified but kept swimming, telling Edna, "Hang in there, you can make it."

Edna and Amanda did make it safely to shore, and Edna was taken to a local hospital where she recovered.[3]

Love compels, love reaches out, and love risks all because love is willing to give all. Love overcomes fear.

There is only one remedy, one cure, one solution for sin and the destruction it causes. It's love: that eternal flame, that primordial passion, that unrelenting longing stemming from the heart of God. "Perfect love drives out all fear" (1 Jn 4:18). God's plan of salvation is to bring eternal healing by restoring his perfect love into our hearts and minds, eradicating the survival-of-the-fittest principle from us (Heb 8:10; Rev 12:11). "The law of the Lord is perfect, reviving the soul" (Ps 19:7 NIV 1984). The law of love heals, restores and revives. Our Father of love is calling us back to his arms of love, back to his universe of love, back to his original design—a life of love.

But love doesn't flow where lies about God are retained.

16

When Love Burns Free

Love is the final end of the world's history,
the Amen of the universe.

NOVALIS

The day will come when, after harnessing the winds,
the tides and gravitation, we shall harness for God the energies
of Love. And on that day, for the second time in the history
of the world, man will have discovered fire.

TEILHARD DE CHARDIN

I AM HUNGRY FOR THE TRUTH ABOUT GOD, to experience the fullness of his love, to live a life of love, to be back in his universe of love. I look around at all the pain and suffering in the world and wonder, *Why hasn't Christ returned? What is God waiting for? Why are we still here?* But then I review human history, watch the nightly news and realize how unprepared planet Earth is for God's love, how deeply the lies about God have penetrated.

Love does not flow where lies about God are retained. Our brains cannot be healed until the lies about God are removed. So God waits. He waits for the good news about him to be taken to the world as a witness to all nations, and then his kingdom of love will come. He doesn't want any to perish but all to be saved, so he waits for us—that's right, *us*—to take the truth about him to the world (2 Pet 3:9).

But have we done it? Have we taken the truth about God to the world—or perhaps a counterfeit? In *Recovering the Scandal of the Cross*, Green and Baker note that the predominant Christian picture of God, taken to the world, hasn't been effective in turning hearts to Christ. This is what they observe:

> If, at least to a significant degree, penal substitutionary atonement has been a "culture product" of life in the West, is it any surprise that proclamation of the gospel grounded in this theory has tended to fall on deaf ears in other social worlds? Christian missionaries from the West, armed with this central affirmation of the gospel—namely, the good news that Jesus has come to take away your guilt, that Jesus has been punished for you so that God can declare you not guilty—have often reported their surprise upon discovering the huge populations of the world for whom guilt is a nonissue.[1]

Could it be the Lord waits because the good news about his kingdom of love has yet to go to the world? Could some Christians still have God-concepts that interfere with God's healing plan?

Perhaps you have heard about Edward Fudge and his questions about hell, or Rob Bell's inquiries in *Love Wins*. Perhaps you also heard about the conflict, ridicule and opposition they faced for honestly seeking answers to a very difficult subject. Many struggle with reconciling a God of love with eternal burning in hell. Have you ever had questions about hell? What does God actually do to those who refuse his love?

In most cultures, hell is depicted as a place of torture and punishment. Within Christianity, the most common view of hell is a place of eternal torment, often in flames. Typically, this is presented as inflicted by a wrathful deity to punish unrepentant sinners.

Fortunately, over the last few decades many voices have arisen to question such a teaching. In the 1990s the Anglican church changed its official position on hell from a place of eternal torment to one of annihilation of the wicked, stating that the teaching of eternal torment makes God into a "sadistic monster."[2]

If God is love, and he wants love as a response from us, the traditional teaching of hell requires serious reevaluation. How can God incite love by threatening to burn those who don't love him, either briefly or eternally? Threats violate freedom, which destroys love and incites rebellion. Yet the Scripture is filled with references regarding eternal fire and torment of the unrepentant. How do we make sense of it all?

In this chapter I want to explore the question, "What happens to the unrepentant wicked in the end?" This will not be a historical review of theological positions nor an exploration of cultural hell myths, nor will I seek to do a contextual verse-by-verse biblical exegesis. Instead, I want to offer a view of this subject that meets the criteria for study set down in the introduction of this book. Specifically, that we use all of Scripture (or as many of the texts as we reasonably can in this short chapter), harmonizing it with God's testable laws, the truth about God as revealed in Jesus and our own experience. With this approach, let's see if we can find a reasonable conclusion that is consistent with the inspired record, yet is true to God's testable laws and his character of love.

EVERLASTING BURNING AND CONSUMING FIRE

In searching my Bible for texts on consuming fire, I read: "The sinners in Zion are terrified; trembling grips the godless: 'Who of us can dwell with the consuming fire? Who of us can dwell with everlasting burning?'" (Is 33:14). I know many a preacher who would like me to think the wicked will live forever suffering horribly in the eternal, burning fires. But I kept reading and was totally blown away. In fact, my world turned upside down when I read Isaiah's answer to who will live in the everlasting burnings. Listen to his description: "he who walks righteously and speaks what is right, who rejects gain from extortion and keeps his hand from accepting bribes, who stops his ears against plots of murder and shuts his eyes against contemplating evil"! (Is 33:15 NIV 1984).

I did a double take, then a triple take. The concept was so foreign, so unheralded, that I reread the same passage in several versions of the Bible. What was going on? At first I couldn't make sense of it. I was so steeped in tradition; my mind was so dependent on what others had taught me that I had never really let God's Word speak directly to me. My preconceived ideas had obstructed me from seeing the truth. Therefore, I searched the entire Bible with a new mindset, allowing the evidence I uncovered within its pages to form my conclusions. I still get tingles when I think about what I found.

I discovered that, when God spoke to Moses from within the bush, the bush burned but did not get consumed (Ex 3:2-4; Acts 7:30-36). When God came to Mt. Sinai, his presence was described as a "consuming fire," but the elements did not melt (Ex 24:17). When Solomon's temple was dedicated, the priests couldn't enter because the brightness of God's fiery; glory was too great, but the temple did not burn down (2 Chron 5:14; 7:1-3). I wondered what kept the priests out of the temple? It didn't seem to be heat.

Then I read how Lucifer, before his fall, walked among the "fiery stones" of God's presence (Ezek 28:14, 16). I remembered the millions of angels living in the rivers of fire cascading from God's throne (Dan 7:9-10).

By now, I was getting excited. I kept searching and read about Jesus, prior to his crucifixion, in a body still subject to death, being bathed in fire, yet no harm came to him. His clothes didn't even get scorched (Mt 17:2). I read in Hebrews that "our God is a consuming fire" (Heb 12:29), and remembered a passage in Song of Solomon: "Love is as strong as death, its jealousy unyielding as the grave. It burns like blazing fire, like a mighty flame. Many waters cannot quench love; rivers cannot sweep it away" (Song 8:6-7).

Could this fire—this consuming, purifying, unquenchable fire— be the blazing love of God?

And finally, I was blown away to discover that, in the new heaven and earth, the sun won't even need to shine because God's very presence will provide all the light that's needed (Rev 22:5).

At long last, I saw it. The lie, so long hidden in the recesses of my mind, now stood naked and exposed. How darkened my mind had been! The lie that Satan has foisted on us, which held me and millions like me in fearful bondage, is this: the place you don't want to go, the place you don't want to be, is the place of eternal burning and consuming fire. But, as amazing as it may seem, that place is God's very presence! And the righteous will spend eternity bathed in the flames of his fiery presence.

CHRIST RETURNS

When Christ returns he doesn't come veiling his glory but in the full splendor of his holy, loving, righteous self—brighter than the sun! Rivers of blazing love surging out from him, the earth will be bathed in his glory (Is 6:3)! The righteous will be transformed by the life-giving fires of love, just like Moses was transformed after being in God's presence. He came down off the mountain with his face radiating heavenly fire. But Moses wasn't in pain; he didn't have third-degree burns. His whiskers weren't even singed.

What was literally causing his face to glow like the sun? Incredible, amazing love!

As I was rejoicing in my discovery of this consuming fire that is not harmful but is the fiery love of God, I recalled the Israelites' reaction. When they saw Moses' face, they shrank back and begged him to wear a veil. They couldn't stand the heavenly light (Ex 34:33-35).

That's when it dawned on me: the fire of love is painful only when the mind is not healed. The guilty conscience, the unregenerate heart that prefers lies and selfishness cannot tolerate the light of love and truth. "This is the verdict: Light has come into the world, but people loved darkness instead of light because their deeds were evil" (Jn 3:19).

My search became more intriguing. Not only are the wicked unable to enjoy the fire of God's love, they are actually destroyed by the brightness of Christ's coming (2 Thess 2:8). This was initially confusing. How could this be? How can a fire that doesn't burn up bushes, buildings or faces consume the wicked in the end? What kind of fire is this? Then it hit me. This fire serves two purposes. It glorifies and protects God's people while it cleanses the earth of sin. This incredible fire totally and irreversibly consumes wickedness.

A fire that consumes sin? What is that? The fire with which I am familiar is combustible, which burns material substances, things made out of molecules, like our homes, furniture and books. But sin is not made out of physical matter. Sin is made out of ideas, thoughts, concepts, attitudes, beliefs. At its core, sin is composed of two elements: lies (from Satan, the father of lies—Jn 8:44) and selfishness. Fires of combustion don't destroy ideas. Fires that burn material substances don't consume lies and selfishness.

So, what does consume a lie? The truth! And what does consume selfishness? Love! And the Holy Spirit is the Spirit of both truth and love. Amazingly, when the Spirit fell at Pentecost, they all witnessed streams of fire over each person (Acts 2:3), yet no one got burned. The building didn't burn down; their clothes didn't ignite. It was their hearts and minds that were touched—cleansed—by that fire, the fire of love and truth. Distortions about God were removed; envy, strife and selfishness were burned out. Love blazed in them again! Just as was promised, they were baptized with the Holy Spirit *and with fire*—the fire of love and truth (Mt 3:11)!

SUFFERING IN THE FLAMES

But, if the fires are the fires of truth and love, then why do the wicked suffer when those fires burn freely? "They perish because they refused to love the truth and so be saved" (2 Thess 2:10).

What happens in the minds of those who reject truth and cling to falsehood when the truth of God comes shining through? I've seen it time after time in my patients. They suffer torment of mind, anguish of heart and suffering of psyche. And what happens to those whose hearts are filled with selfishness when the pure, undiluted, love of God comes blazing through? "If your enemy is hungry, feed him; if he is thirsty, give him water to drink [love him] In doing this, you will heap burning coals on his head" (Rom 12:20). What happens in the mind of the unhealed when they meet pure Love and Truth face to face?

I have many patients who, as children, suffered abuse from their parents. During the process of healing, many wish their parents would simply admit what they have done, ask forgiveness or, in some way, acknowledge their transgression. But, sadly, they generally never do. I ask my patients, "What would happen in your mother's mind or father's heart if they were to acknowledge the severe abuse they perpetrated on you? What would they have to deal with? Would there be guilt, shame, remorse, self-loathing, self-disgust, self-hatred to work through and resolve?"

We can never avoid the truth. We can only delay the day we deal with it. We can deal with the truth about ourselves, our histories, our characters, our mistakes here and now, under God's grace, and we can experience forgiveness, healing, restoration, regeneration and, ultimately, eternal life. Or we can delay dealing with the truth, put it off, deny, externalize, project and blame others. But if we don't deal with the truth now, one day when Christ returns, each person will then come face to face with ultimate truth.

What will it be like on that day for that abusive mother, for that sexually deviant father, to look into the mirror of undiluted truth and see their own selves as they really are, no self-distortion, no lies, just the plain truth? What will it be like for such a person to have full awareness of what his actions did to his child? What will it be like to have this truth sear through his mind in front of the entire universe?

There will be terrible suffering in the flames of God's love but not inflicted as an external penalty. That suffering to come will be the unavoidable torture of soul that *unremedied sin inflicts*. When Moses came out from God's presence with love and favor in his heart, the people shrank back seeking to hide from his face; when Christ arrives, he returns with love and favor, but those solidified in the lies about God cannot stand the light of love and truth, and run hiding from his face (Rev 6:15-16).

How God's heart must break to have his children so settled into the lie about him that they can't stand to be in his presence. No wonder God delays his return, longing for more of his children to be ready to meet him.

REVEALING EVIDENCE

This was exciting and mind-boggling all at the same time. I discovered more Bible evidence, revealing that the fire of God's presence consumes sin and not material substances. God demonstrated that the "consuming fire," which destroys the wicked, is not a fire that burns elements. In Leviticus, I read about Aaron's sons who, as priests, brought unauthorized fire before the Lord:

> Aaron's sons Nadab and Abihu took their censers, put fire in them and added incense; and they offered unauthorized fire before the LORD, contrary to his command. *So fire came out from the presence of the LORD and consumed them, and they died before the LORD. . . .* Moses summoned Mishael and Elzaphan, sons of Aaron's uncle Uzziel, and said to them, "Come here; carry your cousins outside the camp, away from the front of the sanctuary." So they came and carried

them, *still in their tunics,* outside the camp, as Moses ordered. (Lev 10:1-2, 4-5, emphasis mine)

The fire of the Lord "consumed" them, yet their bodies weren't charred and their tunics were still intact. Like the men on the road to Emmaus, my heart burned within me as the truth of God's word seared through the long-held distortions in my mind (Lk 24:32).

God doesn't want to lose any of his children; therefore, he is pouring out every agency in his heavenly arsenal to restore his love in us. We are infected with fear and selfishness, wired to watch out for "number one." But God is preparing a people who will be ready to meet him when he comes, ready to walk right into heaven, ready to live in the blazing flames of his love.

Love will replace selfishness in the hearts of the redeemed. They will be changed—like Moses who, at age forty, murdered an overseer, but at age eighty offered his life to save others. Or Paul, who prior to the Damascus road, used coercion, torture, imprisonment, and stoning to get his way, but after walking with Christ, ultimately gave his life for others (Rom 9:3; 2 Cor 7:3). This is much the same way the Bible describes those who are ready to meet Jesus when he appears, who would not shrink from death (Rev 12:11). Fear and selfishness are replaced with pure, other-centered love.

The sun of righteousness is rising. His rays of healing love are shining (Mal 4:2). His final message of merciful truth is dawning. Do you see it? Do you love it? But more importantly, will you choose it? Will you allow the truth to set you free? Will you accept the truth about God as revealed by Jesus? Will you allow the fire of God's love to burn through you as you love others more than yourself?

Listen, I tell you a mystery: We will not all sleep, but we will all be changed—in a flash, in the twinkling of an eye, at the last trumpet. For the trumpet will sound, the dead will be raised imperishable, and we will be changed. For the perishable must clothe itself with the imperishable, and the mortal with immortality. When the perishable has been clothed with the imperishable, and the mortal with immortality, then the saying that is written will come true: "Death has been swallowed up in victory."

"Where, O death, is your victory?

Where, O death, is your sting?" (1 Cor 15:51-55)

For the Lord himself will come down from heaven, with a loud command, with the voice of the archangel and with the trumpet call of God, and the dead in Christ will rise first. After that, we who are still alive and are left will be caught up together with them in the clouds to meet the Lord in the air. And so we will be with the Lord forever. (1 Thess 4:16-18)

What a day that will be when the fire of God's presence burns free! Billions will be transformed by those everlasting flames of love. In the twinkling of an eye, graves will open, loved ones will unite, angel choirs will sing.

Daniel Cicciaro and John White will be friends once more. Laura will be reunited with her mother, never to be parted. Harold will be laughing as he holds his children in his arms once again. Fran will be rejoicing as she is free from all sickness and pain. Desmond Doss will weep with joy as angels bring lost friends to his side. And heroic Marian and Barbie Fisher, radiant in love, shining like the sun, will walk hand in hand with Jesus by the river of life. No more heartache, no more sickness or pain, with eyes wide open and hearts renewed, we shall meet Jesus face to face.

Yet billions of others who preferred lies to truth, darkness to light, will run from God, screaming in mental anguish. They will suffer in heart and be tormented in psyche as they come face to face with the truth about themselves, their histories, the opportunities rejected, the pain and suffering they have caused—in contrast to the total love, grace and goodness of God. It will be a sad rejoicing, a truly "awe-full" cleansing as the flames of love and truth burn free on planet Earth once more.

Then, at some moment in time, the last element of sin will vanish. Evil and evildoers will be no more. And after all have perished from the ravages of unremedied sin, the fires of combustion will mix with God's unveiled glory, the elements will melt in fervent heat, and the earth will be cleansed (2 Pet 3:12). The earth will become a boiling cauldron, a great lake of fire, in which *death* and hell are completely consumed, and all traces of sin and sinners are totally eradicated (Rev 20:14). Death itself is destroyed, and what could possibly destroy death? Would it not be life, the life-giving glory of God's fiery presence, cleansing all deviation from his design for life? Then the earth will be made new, the eternal home of the righteous (2 Pet 3:13).[3]

Love, anchored in the heart of God, is a thread woven through the fabric of all creation; a filament of energy sustaining all things from the minutest atom to the largest sun, the tiniest amoeba to the greatest whale. Soon, very soon, love will "burn like a blazing fire, like a mighty flame. Many waters cannot quench love; rivers cannot wash it away" (Song 8:6-7).

He is longing to return for you and for me, to reconnect us to his eternal circle of love. But he waits, not wanting any to be lost. He waits for you and me to embrace the truth about him, to be renewed to be like him in character, to practice his methods of love and to take the good news about him to the world; then he will come!

If you are you tired of this sick and selfish world, if you long for your heavenly home, if you are eager to be reunited with departed loved ones, then embrace the God who is love. Let his love transform you, and join with me in sharing this healing view of God with the world. For when the gospel of the kingdom of love goes to the entire world, as a witness to all nations, then the end will surely come.

The choice is yours. While we have power over what we believe, what we believe holds power over us too—power to heal and power to destroy. The ultimate question is, What do you believe about God?

Buddha, Jesus and Preparing Your Brain for Eternity

The character of Jesus, we proclaim, provides humanity with a unique and indispensable guide for tracing the development of maturing images and concepts of God across human history and culture. It is the North Star, if you will. . . . For Christians, the Bible's highest value is in revealing Jesus, who gives us the highest, deepest, and most mature view of the character of the living God.

BRIAN McLAREN

I reached in experience the nirvana which is unborn, unrivalled, secure from attachment, undecaying and unstained. This condition is indeed reached by me which is deep, difficult to see, difficult to understand, tranquil, excellent, beyond the reach of mere logic, subtle, and to be realized only by the wise.

BUDDHA

According to a 2007 National Institute of Mental Health survey, use of Eastern meditation practices has steadily increased in the United States since 2002.[1] Multiple scientific studies have documented the health benefits of Eastern meditation, such as reduced heart rate, blood pressure, anxiety and pain after surgery, in addition to improved depression, recovery time from illness, attention, concentration and performance in school.[2]

Over the last several decades, Eastern practices have become increasingly popular in Christian churches too. Professor Johan Malan of the University of Limpopo, South Africa, documents that Hindu and Buddhist meditation practices are actively being promoted within Roman Catholic and various Protestant denominations, including the Dutch Reformed Church in South Africa.[3]

Yet many Christian leaders speak out against such practices. Ted Wilson, president of the General Conference of Seventh-day Adventists, spoke in his 2010 inaugural speech against the emerging-church movement that is embracing mystical meditative techniques under the term "contemplative spirituality": "Stay away from non-biblical spiritual disciplines or methods of spiritual formation that are rooted in mysticism such as contemplative prayer, centering prayer, and the emerging church movement in which they are promoted."[4]

Eastern practices have made strong inroads into modern medicine. Dr. Herbert Benson of Harvard University has documented a meditation technique common in all modern religions, what he calls the "relaxation response." This technique incorporates Eastern practices of focusing the mind, repeating a word or phrase, engaging in rhythmic breathing and gently pushing away unwanted thoughts. The relaxation-response technique is commonly used in many medical settings today. Dr. Andrew Newberg documents positive brain and health effects from a variety of Eastern meditation practices, and even states God is not necessary to the process.[5]

Dr. Newberg further suggests that Jesus and Buddha both reached "enlightenment" due to years of practicing Eastern meditation. In other words, it was a self-directed, self-originating, self-sustaining process of focused meditation, which according to Dr. Newberg, Christ practiced and taught.[6] But did Christ and Buddha really practice the same meditation and accomplish the same end? Are Eastern practices truly beneficial to the human condition, or are they a subtle form of mental anesthesia, providing symptom relief from the anguish of a mind out of balance from God's design, while permitting the disease of sin to advance unchecked?

The answers to these questions are best achieved through the lens of God's law of love. As we discovered in chapter 1, God is love, and when God built his universe, he constructed it to operate in harmony with his nature and character. God's law, then, is the construction protocol on which the universe is built and is the principle of other-centeredness, giving or beneficence that life is designed to operate on (see chapter 1 for examples).

In chapter 2 we discovered that lies believed broke the circle of love and trust, and resulted in fear and selfishness entering humanity. This is the principle of watching out for self at the expense of others, "kill or be killed." In this condition the mind does not operate as God designed. Instead of perpetual peace, love and joy, the mind is dominated by a need to survive, and is driven by fear, insecurity and threat assessment.

It was not only humankind that was changed by sin but this entire world. Creation, as God designed, was in perfect unity with its Creator, operating on the law of love. It was only *after* sin that planet Earth became infected with Satan's principle of self-first, which caused the dual state in which God's law of love and Satan's law of sin and death exist together.

We see this current coexistence of good and evil in the world around us. Plants produce beautiful flowers, fruits and nuts, but also thorns, thistles and poisons. The rains refresh the earth, yet storms destroy. Despots can murder millions yet love their families, which is the manifestation of our conflicted hearts, filled with fear and self-ishness yet also built to love. Christianity itself teaches our internal dualism with its battle between the spiritual and carnal natures.

Eastern religions teach a cosmic dualism of an *eternal* existence of good and evil in which both good and evil are required for balance in the universe—the yin and yang. As Buddhist Lama Anagarika Govinda explained: "Thus, good and bad, the sacred and the profane, the sensual and the spiritual, the worldly and the transcendental, ignorance and enlightenment, samsara and nirvana, etc., are not absolute opposites, or concepts of entirely different categories, but two sides of the same reality."[7] *This is Satan's hope,* for good and evil to exist together eternally. Selfishness, being out of harmony with God's design for life, has caused our dual state and is the source of our fear of death. Eastern mystics experience the sin-induced fear of death, but accepting the faulty premise of the *eternal* coexistence of good and evil, they do not seek deliverance from evil with its ever-present fear of death. This leaves them with only one of two possible options:

1. Consignment to eternal cycles of rebirth into higher or lower realms dependent on one's karma

or

2. Escape—transcendence—of both good and evil through Eastern meditation

We can trace the motivational basis for Eastern meditation to Buddha, who when tormented by the fear of death, finally found peace in meditation where he transcended both life and death, good and evil, and experienced what the East calls nirvana, satori or enlightenment—and what Christians, using the same practices, call the God Encounter.[8] Eastern philosophies seek to escape the anxiety of our dual state by ascending, through meditation, to another "realm." In Hinduism and Buddhism, this realm is described as a "nondual state" in which one feels unity with the cosmos and one another. Thus, in the brain of the practitioner of Eastern meditation, the torment of being in a dual state is avoided by a self-imposed, artificial euphoria and transient disconnect from individual reality. Yet the actual condition of selfishness and fear, existing in the character of the Eastern practitioner, is not changed, as no intervention is made to confront and overcome it. In other words, Eastern practices create an illusion in which one feels as if they are healed and transformed into a nondual, unified, healthy state, when in actuality they remain infected with fear and selfishness. Their condition remains out of harmony with God's design and thus terminal.

LEFT AND RIGHT BRAIN

The brain is divided into left and right hemispheres, connected by a superhighway of high-speed brain cables called the corpus callosum. The two hemispheres of the brain have different general functions but are designed to work together in a balanced and complementary way. When our brain hemispheres become imbalanced, problems can arise.

One day, Jill Bolte Taylor, a neuroanatomist and researcher in the Harvard department of psychiatry, had a stroke in her left-brain hemisphere. The blood clot that the surgeons removed was the size of a golf ball. During the time when her left-brain was hemorrhaging and its function impaired, her right-brain dominated her brain function, and she experienced nirvana—a state of euphoric oneness with the cosmos and loss of individuality. After her recovery she said:

> Right here, right now, I can step into the consciousness of my right hemisphere, where we are. I am the life-force power of the universe. I am the life-force power of the 50 trillion beautiful molecular geniuses that make up my form, at one with all that is. Or, I can choose to step into the consciousness of my left hemisphere, where I become a single individual, a solid, separate from the flow, separate from you. I am Dr. Jill Bolte Talyor: intellectual neuroanatomist. These are the "we"

inside of me. Which would you choose? Which do you choose? And when?[9]

The brain is a bioelectric organ, which means it has not only chemical signals but also electrical ones. And changing electrical activity in the brain can alter hemispheric dominance. When the brain circuits fire together in different ways, they create different patterns of electrical signals. The electrical signals of the brain, or brain waves, are classified into four general categories: alpha, beta, theta and delta waves. Alpha waves occur when the brain is resting or during REM sleep, the dream state. When we are awake, reading, giving a speech, engaged in focused activity, thinking or problem solving the brain is producing beta waves. Theta brain waves occur when one "zones out," daydreams or allows the mind to freely wander. And delta waves occur in deep sleep, the nondream state.

Eastern meditation techniques increase the frequency of alpha and theta waves, suppressing beta waves and causing increased secretion of a brain chemical called dopamine (which enhances visualization), provoking a predominance of right-brain activity and altering one's entire consciousness.[10] This would cause one to feel a loss of self-awareness, a feeling of unity with the cosmos, more intense mental imagery, and less awareness of time and space. It would also reduce one's ability to discern evidence-based truths.

While practicing Eastern meditation, a Christian's mind is similarly overwhelmed. But Christians practicing this type of meditation are taught that it is all right—as long as one repeats an incidental mantra, like "Jesus have mercy on me," as if this tiny gesture of acknowledgment could overcome the flood of neural phenomena and would magically legitimize it as Christian. Unfortunately, such meditation practices result in an imbalanced brain, with increased right-sided dominance and the subsequent loss of reason, loss of clear thinking and loss of individuality.[11]

The Bible tells us that the Holy Spirit is the Spirit of both truth and love (Jn 14:17; Gal 5:22; 1 Jn 4:8). Truth is comprehended via the left hemisphere of the brain, whereas our sense of unity, oneness and relational connectedness is experienced in the right side of our brains. Biblical meditation, rather than focusing the mind on nothingness, emptying the mind or chanting repetitive mantras, always focuses on some substantive aspect of God and his character of love. Note the focus of biblical meditations:

> Do not let this Book of the Law depart from your mouth; meditate on it day and night, so that you may be careful to do everything written in it. (Josh 1:8 NIV 1984)

> But his delight is in the law of the LORD,
>   and on his law he meditates day and night. (Ps 1:2 NIV 1984)

> Within your temple, O God,
>   we meditate on your unfailing love. (Ps 48:9 NIV 1984)

> I meditate on your precepts
>   and consider your ways. (Ps 119:15 NIV 1984)

> Let me understand the teaching of your precepts;
>   then I will meditate on your wonders. (Ps 119:27 NIV 1984)

> I lift up my hands to your commands, which I love,
>   and I meditate on your decrees. (Ps 119:48 NIV 1984)

All through Scripture it is the same. God calls us to meditate *on his law of love*, which is an expression of his character of love. This is no empty, mindless, thoughtless meditation, but a contemplative, deeply reflective meditation on the beauty of our infinite God and his methods of love. Such meditation requires the balanced engagement of both right and left hemispheres. Such balance not only results in greater health and peace but also growth in Christlikeness. In his book *Anatomy of the Soul*, Dr. Curt Thompson puts it nicely:

> Neuroscience research has discovered that people with a rea-

sonable balance and level of helpful integrated communi-
cation between the different areas of their brains tend to have
reduced anxiety and greater sense of well-being. In other words,
they have put themselves in the position to be available for the
Holy Spirit to create those very characteristics that we so long
to take root in us: love, joy, peace, patience, kindness, goodness,
faithfulness, gentleness, and self-control.[12]

In order to experience the fullness of both truth and love we must
have the activity balanced in both hemispheres of our brains balanced. We must guard against attacks that obstruct the experience of
truth and love.[13]

Our left brain is attacked within Christianity by false ideas about
God's law, with subsequent distorted views of God as a vengeful, punishing tyrant, which incites fear. And sadly, many Christians, rather
than reevaluating their view of God, instead turn to Eastern meditation to calm their chronically active fear circuits. But Eastern meditation inactivates the left brain through meditations designed to shut
it down and so pursue an emotional, transcendental experience.

Interestingly, Newberg's brain research on practitioners of Eastern
meditation would support the conclusion that Eastern meditation im-
balances the brain, contributing to a false sense of reality. The thalamus
is the brain's central hub for data processing. All information (moods,
thoughts, sensations) passes through the thalamus as it is being routed
to its ultimate neural destination. The thalamus also gives us a sense of
what is and isn't real. Subjects who had practiced Eastern meditation
for more than ten years were found to have an imbalance in the activity of the thalamus. This would cause them to feel as if nirvana and
their state of unity with their higher power were real. According to
Newberg, "The thalamus makes no distinction between inner and
outer realities, and thus any idea, if contemplated long enough, will
take on a semblance of reality. Your belief becomes neurologically
real, and your brain will respond accordingly."[14]

Thus we find that Eastern meditation, rather than leading a person to a personal friendship with God, actual transformation of character, and overcoming fear and selfishness, instead isolates one from God, fails to transform character, and avoids the reality of the person's terminal condition for transcendental euphoria. Rather than seeking to achieve deliverance from the infection of evil, Eastern mysticism promotes the eternal existence of both good and evil.

JESUS ACHIEVED WHAT BUDDHA COULD NOT

Jesus Christ stands in stark contrast to Buddha. Jesus Christ, rather than seeking to avoid the fear of death, instead confronted, overcame and destroyed death by the exercise of his human brain in perfect self-sacrificing love (2 Tim 1:9-10). Jesus Christ humbled himself to partake of our terminal condition, and in the brain of Jesus Christ, the dual state of love versus fear and selfishness warred it out. Jesus Christ experienced temptation in every way we do, but he did so without sinning (Heb 4:15). And since we know we are tempted by our "own evil desires" (Jas 1:14), we know that in the human brain of Jesus, the principles of love battled the human fear of death with its drive to survive. Jesus' humanity was tempted with powerful human emotions to fear death and to act to save self.

In Gethsemane Jesus Christ experienced terrible, emotional anguish that caused excruciating temptation, leading the Savior to plead, if it were possible, to avoid the cross (Mt 26:36-39). Jesus experienced, in his humanity, the internal pull of our fallen nature, yet unlike Buddha, he did not seek to escape this condition through a meditation-induced state of altered brain function, causing an illusionary euphoria. He instead overcame this powerful fear of death by perfect love for God and humanity—truly, greater love had no one than this (Jn 15:13).

In the humanity of Jesus Christ the dual state brought about by sin was eradicated! Jesus cleansed humanity by eliminating the powerful drive of fear and selfishness when, in love, he voluntarily surrendered to death (Jn 10:17-18). Thus, he rose on the third day in a humanity that he purified and restored to God's original design. For, if at any point along death's approach Christ would have exercised his power to stop death from taking him, he would have acted in self-interest to save self, and humanity would not have been freed from the infection of fear and selfishness.

As a result, each human being is privileged to receive, via the Holy Spirit, all that Christ has achieved. We can experience cleansing of our characters, such that we enter into a genuine, nondual state of unity and oneness with God, in which our hearts are brought into unity with his. We "die to self" and live a new life of love. This is what God is waiting for, a people who have overcome their fear of death through their unity with Christ. Revelation describes this people as those "[who] did not love their lives so much as to shrink from death" (Rev 12:11). Think about that: a people no longer driven by the fear of dying. They no longer live with their drive to survive controlling them. They no longer live focused on protecting self. They live to love God and others.

Biblical conversion is not the process of meditation to calm the fear circuitry, but rather the confrontation and overcoming of fear and selfishness when we follow our Shepherd into the "valley of the shadow of death," in which we die to ourselves and are renewed with hearts of love for others. Eastern meditation is the process of self avoiding fear by the action of self, which promotes a self-serving self. Christian conversion is the surrender of self—not seeking to save self but dying to self, love replacing selfishness. This is a transient time of great anguish and anxiety. It is not a time of peace and avoidance of fear, but rather the time when we stand our ground, through God's grace, to overcome our inherent fear and insecurity (for example, Jacob's night of wrestling, Peter after his denial, David after Nathan confronted him). It is in this anguish, as we confront the truth intelligently, wrestling with our own selfishness and, ultimately, surrendering to Christ, that we experience his love, a supernatural regeneration, a new set of motives and freedom from fear-based living. We are brought not to a universe of eternal good and evil but to unity and oneness with God, who is eternal love, and a future free from fear, suffering, pain and death.

Many Christians struggle to experience this transformation because they have accepted one of two false systems:

1. A system of imposed law, imposed penalties and legal payment, with God as the ultimate source of inflicted pain, suffering and death (eternal dualism), and/or the existence of an eternal burning hell in which humans are tortured forever (eternal dualism), instead of the truth that God is love and is working to rid his universe of fear and selfishness (sin) in order to bring all things back into the unity of love "at-one-ment" with himself.

2. Or a system of Eastern philosophies, also based on the existence of eternal dualism, which have the ability to calm the fear circuitry of the brain in pursuit of oneness, but at the cost of an imbalanced brain that fails to truly be enlightened with truth or to unite with Christ for transformation of character.

Sadly, theologies with false God-concepts—distorted views of God—teach the *eternal* existence of good and evil, either within a being who is both a loving God and the source of inflicted torture and death, or else a universe which contains both heaven and an eternally burning hell. Such theologies fail to free the mind from fear and, therefore, activate inflammatory cascades, damaging brain and body, inciting selfishness and undermining God's plan of salvation.

The Christianity of Jesus Christ is a healing system based on the truth of God's love, perfectly revealed in Christ: "Anyone who has seen me has seen the Father" (Jn 14:9). It is a modality of selflessness and beneficence, in which all things live to love others more than self. Such a system is in harmony with God's design, just the way he constructed his universe to operate, in perfect harmony with his own nature of love.

When we finally remove the distortions of God from our minds, when we finally stop operating on the same dual landscape of Eastern religions with the promotion of the eternal existence of good and evil, when we finally return to the truth of God's design template of love, and enter into that unity of trust with him, then he will not only cleanse our characters but will also come again and cleanse his universe from fear and selfishness. What a day of victory that will be. Unlike the Eastern sages, we will not hide in a self-induced state of meditative euphoria but will live in a universe eternally free of fear and selfishness, a universe united again on God's law of love. Then we can rejoice, "O death, where is thy sting? O grave, where is thy victory?" (1 Cor 15:55 KJV).

Addendum

Putting It All Together —
Simple Steps to a Healthier Brain

The more often a man feels without acting, the less
he will ever be able to act, and in the long run,
the less he will be able to feel.

C. S. LEWIS

WE HAVE EXPLORED much about the human brain and how our beliefs about God affect our mental and physical health. In this addendum I want to put it all together in practical terms and leave you with specific steps to not only experience a healthier brain here and now but also grow in intimacy with God, preparing your mind for eternity with him.

BRAIN CIRCUITS AND MAJOR DEPRESSION

Major depression is a serious mental illness, affecting approximately 5 percent of the U.S. population in any given year. When someone is depressed, there are major alterations in body and brain functions.

While this disorder has many contributing factors, once depressed the brain circuits show a characteristic dysfunction. I want to use this neural circuitry dysfunction as a template to differentiate between healthy and unhealthy activities, and thereby teach methods for maximizing brain health.

In chapter 2 we explored the brain's alarm system. We learned how the alarm causes the classic fight-or-flight response and that, after the initial startle response, the prefrontal cortex (DLFPC) kicks in and, if no threat exists, turns the alarm off.

When people are depressed, the brain circuitry is out of balance. The DLFPC activity is below normal, so people with depression are impaired in their ability to concentrate, focus, think clearly, plan, organize, problem solve and manage life stress. The anterior cingulate cortex (ACC) is also underactive in depression, contributing to a sense of emotional distance from others and to difficulty making decisions. This is why depressed people are often so ambivalent and can't make up their minds.

The orbital and medial frontal cortexes are the parts of the brain that convict of wrong and redirect away from inappropriate behavior. Imagine trying to take your clothes off in the middle of a church service. If you tried such an inappropriate act, the orbital and medial frontal cortexes would start firing excitedly, causing you to experience discomfort, attempting to direct you away from such behavior. If, as you read this, you experience a little discomfort at the thought of such an embarrassing situation, then a ripple of activity just rolled through your orbital and medial frontal cortexes. When depressed, these two areas are overactive. This means a depressed person experiences intense feelings of inadequacy, guilt and a sense that everything they are doing is wrong.

The amygdala, the brain's alarm, is also overactive in depression, causing a constant sense of fear, apprehension, uneasiness, dread or impending doom. And the pleasure center of the brain, the nucleus accumbens, where all pleasure registers, is unresponsive when depressed. So the depressed person experiences an overwhelming sense of gloom, guilt, inadequacy, fear, apprehension, emotional blunting, distance from others, inability to think clearly, difficulty with problem solving, a sense of being overwhelmed, and impairments in decision making—but no pleasure when objectively good events occur.

When a brain is in this state, not only does a person experience overwhelming emotional pain, but the body is also being damaged. As we have discovered throughout this book, chronic fear activates stress pathways and the immune system, and inflammatory factors are released that damage the body.

Such a state is not desirable or healthy. Any activity that moves the brain circuits toward the imbalance that occurs in depression is unhealthy, whereas any activity that moves the circuits toward normal would be healthy. Therefore, any God-concept that chronically activates the brain's fear circuitry will result in damage to brain and body, ultimately increasing selfishness and undermining salvation. By returning to the truth about God, as revealed in Christ, the brain is healed from fear and selfishness.

When we accept the truth about God, as revealed in Jesus, the lies are removed and trust is reestablished. In trust we surrender our lives to God and open our hearts to him. He sends his Spirit to do a supernatural work of regeneration in our hearts as we stay in a daily trust relationship with him. His Spirit is the Spirit of love and truth, and as we experience his love, our fear subsides. Rather than living selfishly, we seek to bless others. We actually make different choices, stemming from new motives, which increases wisdom and insight. This further develops the prefrontal cortex and calms the amygdala. Our fear level falls, and our confidence and peace grows. As we spend time with our God of love, we become more and more like him.

When we stumble and fall into selfishness, our hearts are grieved, and we immediately go to God, sorrowful for our weakness, longing to be free from such feebleness. In that trust relationship, we experience God's forgiveness, grace and renewing presence to lift us up and put us back on track with his methods again. And we grow closer in likeness to our amazing God of love, until the day we see him face to face.

Here are some actions to take to have a healthy brain and relationship with God:

1. Think for yourself. Just as physical therapy only benefits the one who does it, so too, development of the prefrontal cortex requires exercise.

2. Become a lover of truth, hunger for it, develop an attitude that you want to grow in the truth. God is infinite; we are finite. This means there is an infinite amount of new truth to discover and grow in. So we never "arrive" at the truth because truth is always unfolding, and to believe one has "arrived" closes the mind to further advancement. Remain ready to change your beliefs with new evidence that harmonizes all three threads (Scripture, science and experience).

3. Become intimately familiar with God's laws and methods. Look for the law of love in nature; understand and practice the law of liberty. Reexamine your beliefs through the lens of God's natural law and reject the imperial Roman imposed-law construct.

4. Test all theories about God with Scripture (emphasizing the life of Jesus), God's testable laws and experience. Rightly understood, the truth about God will harmonize with all three. Embrace and hold to God's character of love.

5. Based on the evidence of God's supreme trustworthiness and character of love, surrender yourself to him. Start each day by opening your heart and inviting in his Spirit.

6. Meditate daily on God's character of love, an intelligent, truth-filled appreciation, and focus on God, his kingdom of love and his works of creation.

7. Trust God with your life, future and outcomes, trust which can occur only after evidence of God's trustworthiness is understood and experienced.

8. Practice God's methods. Live altruistically, give to others, vol-

unteer, seek to share what God has given to you with others. The way God built his universe, the more you give the more you will receive. Just as the fire hydrant that gives away more water than the garden hose also receives more water than the garden hose; the more love you give, the more you will receive.

9. Actively seek to share the truth about God's kingdom of love with others. Join organizations focused on taking God's love to the world. Start a ministry, lead Bible studies, fellowship with like-minded believers, and demonstrate the power of God's methods to heal and restore.

10. Live in harmony with God's physical design for life. Avoid known toxins and poisons—physical and spiritual—alcohol, tobacco, illegal drugs, theatrical entertainment, violent games, vulgar reading material, ugly and punitive concepts of God.

11. Exercise regularly—physically and mentally. Physical exercise produces powerful anti-inflammatory factors that suppress those damaging cytokines that arise from stress. Exercise also turns on factors in the brain that stimulate new neuronal growth, as well as chemicals that improve mood. Mental exercise activates neural circuits, causing them to grow stronger.

12. Get regular sleep. There are four physical requirements for life: air, water, food and sleep. The brain region first to be impaired by sleep deprivation is the prefrontal cortex. Regular sleep keeps the prefrontal cortex functioning at its best.

13. Live in harmony with God's laws of nature. Eat healthfully, maintain hydration and get a few minutes of sunlight each day. Healthy food provides the brain with the nutrients it needs and provides antioxidants to reduce inflammatory damage. Hydration removes waste and reduces inflammatory factors, and sunlight, without sunburn, actually reduces cancer risk by converting vitamin D into its cancer-fighting form.

14. Forgive; don't hold grudges. Unforgiveness and grudge holding activate the amygdala and thus the inflammatory cascade, which damages brain and body. Grudge holding also keeps one relationally distrustful and on edge, undermining peace and relational health.

15. Resolve guilt. Unresolved guilt activates the amygdala, increasing inflammation and undermining physical and mental health. Guilt also undermines peace, increases insecurity and undermines resolve, resulting in greater vulnerability to manipulation by others.

16. If fear and insecurity tempt you to act against your conscience in order to win human approval, remember to do the following:

    a. Take a mental step away and ask, *What is the truth? What is the right, healthy and reasonable action for me to take?*

    b. Ask yourself if someone who rejects you or becomes angry with you for doing what you believe is right could really be your friend. Do you really want their approval?

    c. Be willing to set other people free to think or feel any way they choose about you. Ask yourself whether, on some level, you are trying to control what they think about you. Are you thinking, *If I do what they want, then they won't be mad at me?* Consider setting them free to think whatever they want. And the beauty of God's law of liberty is, when you set others free to think whatever they choose about you, you have just set yourself free from the pressure of conforming to their opinion.

    d. Remember, love does what is right, healthy and reasonable, because it is so, not because it feels good in the moment. So look beyond the immediate, to the principles of God's kingdom, and apply those principles even if they feel uncomfortable at the moment.

17. Keep your eyes fixed on Jesus. Live confidently in God's goodness, knowing the reality of his law of love, the design for life, with your heart always hopeful for the day of his soon return.

STUDY GUIDE

1

God Is Love

LEARNING THROUGH BIBLE EXAMPLES

1. Read Luke 24:13-32 and describe what happened in this story.

2. What belief changed in this story?

3. What was the basis for the change in this belief?

4. What was the consequence of changing this belief?

5. What does this teach us about how our beliefs are to be formed?

LEARNING THROUGH SCIENCE AND NATURE

I attended a conference at Harvard University on spirituality in medicine that sought to explore the benefits of spirituality on physical health. Speakers at the conference represented a variety of religious groups: Jewish, Catholic, Protestant, Muslim, Christian Science and Mormon, to name a few. One of the main emphases of the seminar was that people were free to believe whatever they wanted and all beliefs should be equally valued. I pointed out that although the freedom to choose one's own beliefs should be valued, not all beliefs are equally healthy. Consider the following scenario, recognizing people are free to believe whatever they choose, but evaluate the various costs and benefits resulting from which belief is actually chosen.

Wanda was admitted to the hospital for severe depression. She was required to wear oxygen at night due to severe lung disease. During my evaluation she disclosed that she smoked two packs of cigarettes per day. When I asked why she smoked, given her lung problems, she stated, "Smoking helps me breathe better."

1. Was Wanda free to believe cigarettes helped her breathe better?

2. What was the consequence for believing this?

3. Does science provide evidence that would demonstrate her belief to be false?

4. What would motivate a person to cling to a belief in the face of contradicting scientific evidence?

5. Consider your beliefs about God, and reflect on the law of love described in chapter 1. Examine God's creation. Where do you find evidence of God's love in nature and science?

LEARNING THROUGH EXPERIENCE

Jerry had a lifelong pattern of exploiting others, bending the rules and manipulating the system. Jerry was a dentist who had recently lost his license for illegally selling narcotic pain prescriptions to make money. Jerry refused to accept any personal responsibility but instead blamed society for having draconian rules on substance use, restricting adults from making their own decisions. He insisted he had done nothing wrong, since he was merely ensuring the drug users (who, he said, would use drugs anyway) got a safe and pharmaceutically clean supply of drugs. Jerry believed he was helping others.

1. What unhealthy beliefs did Jerry have?

2. What consequences did this have for Jerry—both professionally and even spiritually?

3. Can God heal Jerry as long as he holds to such beliefs? Why or why not?

4. What truth might help Jerry?

5. List three examples from your life where you have changed your beliefs. What happened as a result of changing your belief, and what factors led you to change your belief?

2

The Human Brain and Broken Love

LEARNING THROUGH BIBLE EXAMPLES

1. Read Genesis 3:1-6 and describe what happened in this passage.

2. What belief changed in this story?

3. What was the basis for the change in belief?

4. What was the consequence of changing this belief?

5. How could this lie be exposed and the truth retained?

6. Read 1 Samuel 16:7. What does it mean that God looks upon the heart?

7. Now read Hebrews 8:10. What does writing the law on the heart mean?

8. Discuss the difference between external behavior and a heart's motive.

9. What law does God desire to "write" onto the hearts of humankind?

LEARNING THROUGH SCIENCE AND NATURE

1. Describe five healthy activities that result in positive emotional experiences, and identify which principles of God are utilized during these activities.

2. Describe five destructive activities that cause initially positive emotional experiences, and identify which principles of God are being violated during these activities.

LEARNING THROUGH EXPERIENCE

1. Recount two times you have believed a lie.

2. What impact did believing the lie have on you and your relationships?

3. Did love and trust get stronger?

4. How did you discover the lie was a lie?

5. What impact did the truth have on you and your relationships?

6. Recount two times you told a lie.

7. What was that experience like? Did you experience anxiety and stress? Were your relationships impacted?

8. Review the brain circuits in chapter 2 and contemplate the impact that such action has had on your health.

9. What happened when the truth was revealed?

3

The Infection of Fear

LEARNING THROUGH BIBLE EXAMPLES

1. Read Romans 7 and describe what Paul is writing about.

2. What is the source of Paul's turmoil?

3. Does it make a difference to realize that all humans since Adam and Eve have been born infected with fear and selfishness, and that they didn't choose to be this way?

LEARNING THROUGH SCIENCE AND NATURE

1. Science has shown that the mind affects the body and the body affects the mind. List examples from your experience where this has happened.

2. How do illness and fever affect your mood and your ability to think sharply?

3. How do powerful emotions affect your appetite, sleep and energy? Do you ever get aches and pains when you're upset?

4. List three activities you can do or can change in order to improve your physical and mental health.

LEARNING THROUGH EXPERIENCE

1. Identify the fears you struggle with (e.g., fear of abandonment, what others think, getting fat, getting sick, not being loved, failing, finances, not being good enough).

2. How do your fears impact you?

3. What actions do you take as a result of your fears?

4. What beliefs have you developed based on fear?

5. Examine your fear in light of truth, evidence and facts. What lessons can be learned?

6. What principles of God can bring healing? (If you're unsure, don't worry; just keep reading and doing more lessons.)

7. List three of your favorite television programs, and then list the emotions these programs arouse. Compare these emotions, feelings and desires with God's principles, and describe any conflicts you find.

8. Examine the content of the programs you watch, and compare the content with God's principles, methods and motives (see Philippians 4:8).

4

Freedom to Love

LEARNING THROUGH BIBLE EXAMPLES

1. Read Matthew 27:19-54 and describe what happened.

2. Do you believe Jesus was not only man but also God? Did Jesus have the power, if he chose to utilize it, to deliver himself from the cross?

3. What do we learn about Jesus and God based on the fact that he didn't do this?

4. When Jesus was faced with the choice of saving himself by the use of his power or giving humankind the freedom to kill him, what choice did he make?

5. What does this say about the kind of being God is and about God's valuing of freedom?

6. Read Revelation 13:11-17 and describe what is happening.

7. What methods are being employed (pay special attention to verses 16-17)?

8. What differences do you notice between the methods of Christ and the methods of the beast?

9. What implication does this have for your life?

LEARNING THROUGH SCIENCE AND NATURE

In the first decade of the twenty-first century, the news reported how the Taliban treated people under its rule: there were strict regulations on all aspects of one's personal life, including dress, travel, diet and speech. If someone were to choose to become a Christian, they would be executed.

1. If you lived in such a society, how would you react?

2. Which law of God is being violated by such behavior?

3. While the Taliban are an extreme example, describe why no government of the world accurately represents the government of God.

4. Can love be won by the use of might, power, force and coercion?

5. Would you want to live eternally in a universe governed like the Taliban governs?

6. Have you ever heard anything taught within Christianity that would violate God's law of liberty? If so, what?

LEARNING THROUGH EXPERIENCE

1. Describe two examples in your life where you had your liberties violated.

2. How did you react?

3. Did love get stronger or get damaged?

4. What did you do to get your freedom back?

5. If you are currently in a situation where freedoms are being violated (whether it is your freedoms that are being violated or you are violating someone else's), describe what you can do to restore liberty in your life and relationships.

6. Have you ever been worried about what people think of you? (If you have not experienced this, then answer with what you think would happen to someone who was in that situation.)

7. Describe how these feelings can lead to loss of liberty.

8. When you surrender your individuality to the opinions of others, what happens to you?

9. If you know someone who does this regularly, does this type of behavior cause you to admire and respect him or her more?

10. If you set others free to think whatever they want of you, realizing their opinions don't determine reality, what happens to you?

5

Love Strikes Back

LEARNING THROUGH BIBLE EXAMPLES

God created the world to operate on the principle of love. When humankind sinned, the principle of self-first infected creation.

1. Read Exodus 2:11-12. What principle was Moses operating on in this scene?

2. Read Exodus 32:31-32. What principle was Moses operating on in this scene?

3. Read Acts 8:1-3. What principle was Saul of Tarsus practicing in his life?

4. Read 2 Corinthians 12:15. What principle was Paul (formerly Saul) practicing then?

5. Read 1 John 3:16. What principle is being described?

6. Read Revelation 12:11. What character trait is being described here, regarding those who are ready to meet Jesus when he comes?

7. Read Luke 7:36-50 and describe what is happening.

8. What motivated the woman to anoint Jesus' feet?

9. What motivated those who criticized her?

10. What did Jesus say regarding those who are forgiven much?

11. Have you experienced God's forgiveness and love in your life? What affect has this positive or negative experience had on you?

LEARNING THROUGH SCIENCE AND NATURE

The law of love is the principle of outward, other-centered giving, and it emanates from the character of God himself. All creation is designed with this principle as its basic code of operation, the secret on which life is founded. Describe examples of this principle that you can observe in the world around you.

LEARNING THROUGH EXPERIENCE

1. Describe an experience where you acted in love, with a genuine interest in giving to benefit another without any expectation or desire for reward. What happened inside you?

2. Now describe an experience where selfishness dominated your actions, where you were thinking of your needs, desires and wants, forgetting about others. What happened inside of you? Contrast this experience with times when you acted in love; what differences do you observe?

6

Engaging the Battle

LEARNING THROUGH BIBLE EXAMPLES

1. Read 2 Samuel 13:1-15. When verse 1 says Amnon "fell in love," do you think this was love?

2. What was the motivation for his action?

3. After acting on lust, does fear go up or down? What does fear lead one to do?

4. If you are attracted to someone who is not interested in you and you act with genuine love, what action will you take?

LEARNING THROUGH SCIENCE AND NATURE

1. Imagine that you've found an injured sparrow. You have a desire to rescue it, but as you approach to save it, the bird does all in its power to flee.

2. What motivates the bird to act this way?

3. What lessons are there in this scenario regarding how we act toward God in our spiritual sickness?

4. Does fear lead to greater openness and trust, or greater secrecy and caution?

LEARNING THROUGH EXPERIENCE

1. When you have sinned, do you or have you ever struggled with fear of God?

2. What helped you overcome that fear in order to open your heart to him?

3. What would you say to someone who is struggling with guilt and too afraid of God to open her heart to him?

4. If you became sick from doing IV drugs and had a high fever, would you be afraid to go to the doctor or would you want to go? Would you want to go see a judge? Does it make a difference in opening our hearts to God if we see him as our heavenly physician instead of a cosmic judge?

7

Love Stands Firm

LEARNING THROUGH BIBLE EXAMPLES

1. Read Judges 16:6-22. How would you describe the relationship depicted here?

2. Was this a love-based relationship?

3. In Judges 16:16, Delilah accuses Samson of not loving her. What do you make of this?

4. If Samson did love her with a godly love, what would he have told her? So why did he tell her what he did? Did Delilah love Samson?

5. Does godly love ever require a person to violate his or her conscience?

6. Read 2 Samuel 11:2-16 and describe what happened.

7. What motivated David to pursue Bathsheba? Were his actions based on love?

8. Once she became pregnant, how did David respond?

9. What motivated David's actions?

10. What was the consequence for David?

11. What is the lesson from this for when we let fear override love?

LEARNING THROUGH SCIENCE AND NATURE

In today's society, people turn to many sources to alleviate fear in decision making—astrology, fortune-tellers, witchcraft, friends, powerful feelings, religious leaders, alcohol, drugs and so on.

1. Which sources for alleviating fear are reliable, and which ones are unreliable?

2. What makes a resource reliable?

3. Is there a difference between "claims" and "evidence"? Which one is more trustworthy?

4. How would you describe genuine, godly love? Is godly love reliable or unreliable? Is it a feeling, more than that, or something else?

5. In Gethsemane, did Jesus experience powerful feelings? What was the emotional tenor of his feelings? Did he act on those feelings or take an action contrary to what the feelings wanted? Did Jesus choose to act in harmony with love? If so, what does this tell us about love and emotions?

6. Review the scientific studies at the end of chapter 1, which document the impact volunteerism has on health. What do studies like those tell us about love?

LEARNING THROUGH EXPERIENCE

1. List three examples of situations where you have been tempted by fear or insecurity.

2. How did you choose whether to give in to the fear?

3. What were the consequences when you went with fear?

4. What were the consequences when you did what you knew was right and loving, despite the fear?

5. What choice would you make today, and why?

8

Changing Our View of God

LEARNING THROUGH BIBLE EXAMPLES

1. Read John 4:4-29 and describe what transpired here.

2. How did Jesus initiate contact with this woman?

3. Why did he ask her to do something for him rather than simply proclaiming the truth?

4. How did Jesus bring her to have confidence in him?

5. Do you think Jesus was breaking down preconceived ideas she held about God? If so, describe how.

6. What did Jesus' actions reveal to us about God?

LEARNING THROUGH SCIENCE AND NATURE

1. Many people believe that there is no God, that nature reveals only natural forces at work. What evidence can you provide that supports the existence of God and his character of love?

2. We cannot demonstrate either the Big Bang or Creation in a lab experiment, but we can examine the assumptions both theories rest on. Examine each of the assumptions below and then list tests or experiments we can do today to demonstrate whether the various assumptions are true or not. Which assumptions are and are not scientifically valid, based on what can be demonstrated today?

- Evolution: something came from nothing
- Creation: something came from something

- Evolution: life comes from nonliving matter
- Creation: life comes from living matter

- Evolution: complex things come from chaos without any intelligent input
- Creation: complex things come from chaos with intelligent input

LEARNING THROUGH EXPERIENCE

1. List two beliefs about God you have changed during the course of your life.

2. Discuss the basis for the change in belief, as well as the impact on your life when the belief changed.

3. Mark was angry with God and, despite being raised in a conservative Christian home, no longer attended church. Ever since the death of his unborn child, he no longer believed God cared. He concluded that if God were all-powerful and all-loving, he wouldn't sit by idly and let children be sick and die.

   If Mark were your spouse or friend, what might you say to him?

4. What Bible examples can you give that deal with this issue?

5. How does Zechariah 4:6—which says, "'Not by might nor by power, but by my Spirit,' says the LORD"—apply?

6. God has all power, yet he prefers to win people rather than coerce people. How does this truth impact your life?

9

The Power of Truth

LEARNING THROUGH BIBLE EXAMPLES

1. Read 1 Kings 13:11-25. What is being described here?
2. Is the old prophet a false prophet?
3. Did the old prophet lie?
4. What is the lesson? Are we responsible for the truth God has presented to us, regardless of what some other person—including one claiming to be speaking for God—might say?
5. Read John 8:32. What does this mean?
6. List three biblical examples of truth setting people free.

LEARNING THROUGH SCIENCE AND NATURE

History is replete with accounts of doctors utilizing treatments that not only failed to help but actually harmed. For more than two millennia, physicians practiced bleeding and leeching to drain evil humors. George Washington, after falling ill, had half his body's blood drained, certainly accelerating his demise.[1]

Tobacco was used by doctors for centuries to treat a variety of medical illnesses, including ulcers, polyps, skin lesions, headaches, respiratory problems and diseases of the glands.[2] In the nineteenth century, doctors used a variety of poisons, such as opium, quinine, arsenic, calomel (mercury), antimony and strychnine to treat a broad range of conditions.[3] They called these toxins "medicines."

1. What do these examples tell us about "secular" truth? Is it progressive, unfolding and increasing over time?

2. Is it healing to embrace and apply the truth once it is understood?

3. What about spiritual truth? Is our understanding of God increasing over the centuries, or are we stuck with antiquated concepts that in some instances are no healthier than leeching?

4. Identify examples of unfolding spiritual truth.

LEARNING THROUGH EXPERIENCE

1. Examine three decisions you regret most in your life. What would you do differently if you could? How many of those decisions were made based on truth, and how many were made either because you believed a lie or you knew the truth at the time but chose to ignore it?

2. What does your own experience tell you about the power of truth?

---

[1]V. Vadakan, "The Asphyxiating and Exsanguinating Death of President George Washington," *The Permanente Journal* 8, no. 2 (Spring 2004); Gilbert R. Seigworth, "Bloodletting Over the Centuries," *New York State Journal of Medicine* (December 1980), www.pbs.org/wnet/redgold/basics/bloodlettinghistory.html.
[2]James Grehan, "Smoking and 'Early Modern' Sociability: The Great Tobacco Debate in the Ottoman Middle East (Seventeenth to Eighteenth Centuries)," *The American Historical Review* 5, no. 3 (2006); S. A. Dickson, *Panacea or Precious Bane: Tobacco in Sixteenth Century Literature* (New York: New York Public Library, 1954); J. E. Brooks, *The Mighty Leaf: Tobacco Through the Centuries* (Boston: Little, Brown, 1952); G. G. Stewart, "A History of the Medicinal Use of Tobacco, 1492-1860," *Med Hist.* 11, no. 3 (1967): 228-68; A. Charlton, "Medicinal Uses of Tobacco in History," *Journal of the Royal Society of Medicine* 97, no. 6 (June 2004): 292-96.
[3]J. Haller, *American Medicine in Transition, 1840-1910* (Urbana: University of Illinois Press, 1981), p. 67.

10

The Truth About Sin

LEARNING THROUGH BIBLE EXAMPLES

1. Read Isaiah 1:10-18. In these verses, God berates the people of Israel in an effort to alert them to how far they are from his ideal. He even refers to them as Sodom and Gomorrah. But in these verses, what specific activities is God upset with them for doing?

2. Who told the people to offer animal sacrifices, to come to the temple, to observe the sabbath and to keep the feast days? If they were doing the activities God had instructed them to do, then why was he upset with them?

3. Read Isaiah 1:13 closely. God tells the people to "stop bringing meaningless offerings." What does it mean to bring a "meaningless" offering?

4. Were the various religious observances and rituals God instructed the people to participate in capable of curing humanity's sin?

5. According to Hebrews 9:9, 14 and 10:2, why were the rituals not able to cure humanity of sin?

6. What insight does this give as to where sin occurs?

7. Read John 6:53-59. What is being described here? Is Jesus being literal or metaphorical?

8. When you think about the "blood of Jesus," what comes to mind?

9. Where did Jesus say his blood is to be applied? What does this mean?

10. Could it mean we are to internalize Christ into our hearts? Does this give any insight regarding the truth about sin?

LEARNING THROUGH SCIENCE AND NATURE

Imagine you have a child, and during your child's youth, you have taught him or her to live in harmony with the laws of health—to not smoke, to eat right, to exercise, not to do drugs or alcohol, to drink plenty of water, etc. However, once your child is grown and on his or her own, your child rebels, "finally free from all those rules." Your child begins to smoke, do drugs, drink heavily, never exercise and eat only junk food.

1. What would happen, and how would you respond?

2. Would you stop loving your child?

3. Would you inflict diseases, sicknesses or death on your child to make him or her pay for disobeying what you taught?

4. Would you try to reach out to your child to redeem, heal and restore?

5. If your child became sick with liver failure and cancer from violating all the laws of health, how would you feel?

6. What would you do if you had a cure for your child, but your child refused the cure? Would you kill your child? Would you let your adult child make his or her own choice?

7. What lessons can we learn from this example about sin and how God deals with us?

LEARNING THROUGH EXPERIENCE

1. List three examples in your life when you knowingly did something wrong. What happened to you after each action?

2. Did you have more peace or less? Did your loss of peace come from an external or internal source? What does this indicate about what sin does to the sinner?

3. If you didn't immediately correct your mistake, what happened to your thinking? Were you tempted to make excuses or blame others? What does this mean in regard to critical thinking and the ability to examine evidence without bias?

4. Did your relationships get healthier and more harmonious? Why or why not?

5. What action was necessary to heal the damage and find peace again?

6. What happens to people who refuse to accept responsibility for their mistakes and refuse to experience a change in their heart attitudes through God's grace?

11

Enlarging Our View of God

LEARNING THROUGH BIBLE EXAMPLES

1. Read Judges 6:36-39. What did Gideon ask God to do?

2. While we believe that God is the one acting in this exchange with Gideon, do you think Satan has the ability to make a fleece wet and the ground dry? Do you think a human being could produce such an event? If so, describe ways a human could put a dry fleece on wet ground or a wet fleece on dry ground.

3. Both times God granted Gideon's request. Do you find this evidence to be the most reliable God can give? Is this evidence easily counterfeited?

4. What does it say about God that he is willing to meet people where they are and provide evidence they need?

5. Read Genesis 18. How did Abraham respond to God when God told him he was going to destroy the cities on the plain?

6. Should Abraham have said, "God said it; who am I to question God?"

7. What does it say about God that Abraham could question him as he did?

8. What does this imply regarding God's desire for us to speak our minds to him?

LEARNING THROUGH SCIENCE AND NATURE

Jesus used many parables from nature. Pick one and explain how the example from nature reveals God and his character of love.

LEARNING THROUGH EXPERIENCE

Describe an experience in your life when you struggled to understand God and his actions.

1. Based on concepts from chapter 11, what are some possible ways to understand that event that are in harmony with God's character of love?

2. Have you told God what is really on your mind? Have you expressed your frustration and heartache to him? If not, consider telling him exactly what your burden is, and then ask him to help you find the truth.

12

The Judgment of God

LEARNING THROUGH BIBLE EXAMPLES

1. Read Psalm 34:8 and John 17:3. What do you think these texts mean?

2. Do they indicate anything regarding the necessity of making judgments of God?

3. Does God want us to examine him and the evidence he has provided in order to make a decision, a judgment, on whether we can trust him?

4. Read Luke 24:13-32. Did this event occur before or after Jesus' resurrection?

5. Did Jesus use might and power to influence their decision?

6. What method did Jesus use?

7. Why was it necessary for Jesus to utilize the evidence of Scripture and his own life?

8. What does this tell us about God and how he relates to us?

LEARNING THROUGH SCIENCE AND NATURE

1. What testable laws can you identify that demonstrate God is trustworthy?

2. Consider forensic science. Do people who are innocent of any crime need to fear the full and accurate disclosure of forensic evidence?

3. What evidence can you cite that confirms God is completely trustworthy? (Make a distinction between claims/proclamations, testable evidence and recorded historical events.)

LEARNING THROUGH EXPERIENCE

Think of one or two people in your life who you genuinely, completely trust with your life—people you know would rather die than harm you.

1. Why do you trust this person or these people?

2. What evidence do you have of their trustworthiness? Is your trust based on claims?

3. Did you have to work to trust them, or did trust naturally result from your experience with them?

4. If these people who you have found to be trustworthy told you something they did that you didn't have evidence for, would you believe them? If so, does that mean your faith in them is without evidence? Or has your faith in them been established on previous evidence?

5. Would these people, who are trustworthy, be offended if evidence became available that supported what they had previously told you—and you examined it?

6. Would examining the evidence for a genuinely trustworthy person undermine trust or strengthen it?

7. What do you believe God wants in regard to your judgment of him—for it to be evidence based or based on claims?

13

In the Brain of Christ

LEARNING THROUGH BIBLE EXAMPLES

1. Read Matthew 26:36-42. What is being described?

2. What emotions did Jesus experience?

3. Did these emotions tempt Jesus? If so, what did they tempt him to do?

4. According to James 1:13, divinity cannot be tempted, so where did these powerful emotional temptations come from?

5. In conjunction with Hebrews 2:14, what does this reveal regarding Jesus' humanity?

6. Read John 10:17-18. What is Jesus telling his disciples about his nature?

7. What principle is being evidenced in this passage?

8. When comparing the emotions Jesus experienced in Gethsemane with the principle expressed in this passage, what two antagonistic principles are revealed?

9. What are the implications for what was happening in the decision-making part of Jesus' brain?

LEARNING THROUGH SCIENCE AND NATURE

1. Examine the laws of health. Can a doctor heal a patient in violation of the laws of health, or do all healing interventions work to restore a person back into harmony with the laws

of health? Give three examples of medical interventions that restore a person to harmony with the laws of health.

2. Could God heal and restore humankind to his original design in violation of his law? Or would man's salvation require being restored to harmony with God's law, his design for life?

3. Examine again the law of love as described in chapter 1, then discuss how Christ acted in perfect harmony with God's law. What is the implication for humanity?

LEARNING THROUGH EXPERIENCE

1. As a parent, have you ever had to use force in dealing with your child? Did you prefer to act this way? If not, then why did you do it? Does loving discipline restrain and even inflict pain, if necessary, to save and protect?

2. Did your heart rejoice in the moments when you acted in such ways? Or did your heart long for your child to grow up so that such interventions would never be necessary again?

3. What do you believe is God's attitude toward the exercise of force in relationship with us?

4. What conclusion do you draw if Jesus is the filter through which you see God?

5. Have you surrendered your life to Jesus Christ and asked for the Holy Spirit to enter into your heart?

   • If not, what prevents you from doing so? Is the evidence of God's trustworthiness sufficient to earn your trust? If not, what is needed to win your trust?

   • If so, what has been your experience since surrendering your heart to him? Have you experienced anything like new motives, peace, increasing insight and wisdom, or increasing love for others? If so, where do you think such transformational power comes from?

14

Forgiveness

LEARNING THROUGH BIBLE EXAMPLES

1. Read Genesis 37:23-28 and 45:3-7. Describe the situation—who was offended and who did the offending?

2. What was necessary for reconciliation to take place?

3. Who forgave? What enabled him to forgive?

4. Who repented and how was the repentance demonstrated?

5. Would reconciliation have occurred without both repentance from the offenders and forgiveness from the offended?

6. Read Genesis 34 and describe the situation. Who was offended and who did the offending?

7. What was necessary for reconciliation to take place?

8. Who repented and who forgave?

9. Who didn't forgive?

10. What happened as a consequence of unforgiveness?

LEARNING THROUGH SCIENCE AND NATURE

Recently I had the privilege of meeting Kent Whitaker. In December 2003, Kent, his wife and their two sons, Bart and Kevin, went out to dinner to celebrate Bart's upcoming graduation from college, where they gave Bart a $4,000 Rolex as a graduation gift. After dinner, Kevin, the younger brother, drove the family home.

As they approached the house, Bart turned back to the car to get his cell phone. But when the rest of the family entered the house, a masked gunman shot and killed Kevin and his mom. Since Kent was the third to step into the doorway, he was shot in the chest, but survived. It turned out that Bart had arranged to have his family shot and killed so that he could inherit the family money. Bart was arrested and put on trial for murder, with the prosecutor seeking the death penalty.

Kent publicly forgave his son and asked the prosecutor not to seek the death penalty. However, the prosecutor sought the death penalty anyway, and Bart was found guilty and sentenced to death. Throughout the trial of his son, Kent was consistently loving toward Bart, visiting him regularly in prison and openly forgiving him for what he did. His son eventually said, "If you can still love me and forgive me for all I have done, then I believe God can also." Bart gave his life to Christ in prison. Kent states that, although he has lost his wife and younger son on this earth and will lose Bart too, he has peace knowing that through all of this Bart will now be with them in heaven. Their family will be together for eternity.

1. How does this story reveal the two antagonistic principles of God's love versus fear and selfishness?

2. How does Kent's forgiveness contradict the worldly principle of "me first"?

3. What is the impact of Kent's forgiveness? Did it bring healing or further hostility?

4. How might you have responded if you were in Kent's position?

5. What enabled Kent to forgive his son?

6. How is love involved in forgiving others?

Every day the news is filled with Israeli and Palestinian violence — a suicide bombing on a metro bus, a retaliatory airstrike, followed by another bombing, followed by more military action—and the cycle seems to have no end.

7. How could God's principles of forgiveness change this situation?

8. What prevents people from experiencing and practicing God's methods of forgiveness?

LEARNING THROUGH EXPERIENCE

1. Carefully examine yourself and your personal relationships, and list any people who you have offended and have never sought forgiveness. Also list any "sins" you have never repented of (this could include offenses against God).

2. Would you like to heal? Make the choice to forgive, and ask God to help you forgive.

   • Do this for every unresolved issue in your heart.

   • Seek God, tell him of your sorrow for any mistakes you may have made, and accept his forgiveness.

   • Forgive yourself.

   • Then seek God's wisdom on how to heal and repair any damage you may have caused. Learn from the experience, and implement godly changes so that you don't continue to repeat the same unhealthy choices over again.

   • Finally, seek to repair any damage you may have caused, always keeping in mind not to actually cause more injury in the process (e.g., if you had an affair years ago with a person who is now deceased, it would not be loving or helpful to go to the deceased person's spouse and "confess and ask forgiveness"—as this would harm the innocent spouse by planting hurt into his or her heart).

15

When Good Prevails

LEARNING THROUGH BIBLE EXAMPLES

1. Second Corinthians 5:17-20 states:

    Anyone who is joined to Christ is a new being; the old is gone, the new has come. All this is done by God, who through Christ changed us from enemies into his friends and gave us the task of making others his friends also. Our message is that God was making all human beings his friends through Christ. God did not keep an account of their sins, and he has given us the message which tells how he makes them his friends.

    Here we are, then, speaking for Christ, as though God himself were making his appeal through us. We plead on Christ's behalf: let God change you from enemies into his friends! (GNT)

    What does this text describe Christ doing with his enemies?

2. Is this different that what humans typically do with their enemies?

3. What happens when enemies are turned into friends?

4. How does Christ achieve this?

5. Read Revelation 12:11. What is this text describing about the character and motives of the people of God?

6. Is this description of people before or after the second coming of Christ?

7. What enables people to experience such love as described in this verse and shown in this chapter?

LEARNING THROUGH SCIENCE AND NATURE

Many humanists claim that giving in to hedonistic desires, as long you're not violating the human rights of another, is perfectly healthy.

1. What evidence can you cite that hedonistic self-indulgence is harmful?

2. From what you have learned in this book about the brain, what part of the brain is responsible for godly love?

3. From what part of the brain do selfish drives arise, and which part of the brain is strengthened by hedonistic indulgence?

4. What implication would this have regarding our ability to exercise godly love toward others?

LEARNING THROUGH EXPERIENCE

1. Consider the persons you respect the most and why. Do they demand their rights, or are they willing to surrender their rights to help others?

2. Describe an event when someone acted selflessly or sacrificially for you. What affect did that have on you?

3. Describe an event in your life when love empowered you to overcome fear. What is the lesson from that experience?

When Love Burns Free

LEARNING THROUGH BIBLE EXAMPLES

Review the following biblical texts: Exodus 3:2-4; 34:29-35; 2 Chronicles 5:14; 7:1; Isaiah 33:14-15; 2 Thessalonians 2:10; Hebrews 12:29.

1. What do these text teach about the source of "consuming fire"?

2. Many good-hearted people have been taught that God says, "I am love and only want you to love me. But if you don't I will be forced to torture and kill you (burn you in hell)." What is the problem with this position?

3. What law of God does this position violate?

4. If this were true, what kind of being would God be?

5. If this were true, could you trust God?

LEARNING THROUGH SCIENCE AND NATURE

Review the evidence of God's law of liberty as described in chapter 4. Test it in a variety of situations.

1. Are you confident of its reality?

2. Where does this law originate?

3. Can love exist without freedom?

4. What impact does it make on our understanding of God's attitude toward the wicked in the end?

5. Reexamine the difference between natural law and imposed law, as described in chapter 13. Which type of law is God's government built on?

6. Contrast the differences between violations of natural law and imposed law. Which view more accurately represents God?

LEARNING THROUGH EXPERIENCE

1. If your spouse said, "Love me or I will beat you to death," how would you respond?

2. When you are threatened, do you experience greater love and trust? Or do love and trust get damaged?

3. Who wants to damage your love and trust in God?

The president of Iran stated that the twelfth imam (the Islamic Savior) would soon appear, and when he comes he will use his great power to kill all the infidels (Jews, Christians, and anyone else who doesn't follow the way of Islam). Let's change this statement to read, "Jesus is soon to come and will use his great power to kill all who don't believe in him," and then answer the following questions:

4. Is there any significant difference between the two statements?

5. Do the "gods" represented in the two statements differ in any significant way?

6. If you believe Jesus will use great power to inflict pain, suffering and death on people, what reaction does that engender?

7. List the new truths about God you have learned while reading this book.

8. Describe how these truths have affected your relationship with God, and if you appreciate God, tell him how much and why.

Then tell three people about the truths you have learned, and how it has affected your relationship with God.

17

Buddha, Jesus and Preparing
Your Brain for Eternity

LEARNING THROUGH BIBLE EXAMPLES

1. Read Psalm 23. Consider this psalm a description of the experience of salvation, being led by our Shepherd through a valley where we "die to self" for his righteousness's sake in order to restore our souls. Then describe the meaning of each verse in this transformational experience.

2. What does it mean that, at the end of this journey, we dwell in the house of the Lord forever?

The Bible records the life of Jesus. It records his miracles, including his control over winds and storms, walking on water, turning water to wine, healing the sick and raising the dead. Christ himself stated that the Father had put all things under his power, and then Jesus got up and washed his disciples' feet (Jn 13:3-5). At the cross, Christ had the power to come down and slay his abusers, but instead, he chose to not use his power to save himself nor to hurt those bent on killing him.

3. What does this evidence say about the kind of person Jesus is?

4. When you see someone being abused and choosing to restrain themselves, not striking out against the abuser when they clearly

could, does that increase your faith in how they would treat you?

5. Jesus said that if we have seen him we have seen his Father—they are one. When you think of the Father, do you take the evidence Christ has revealed about his character and see God in that very light?

6. Can you trust a God like this?

LEARNING THROUGH SCIENCE AND NATURE

Review the evidence of Jesus' accomplishments in Scripture, highlighted in chapter 13, and then discuss the differences between what Jesus accomplished and what Buddha did.

LEARNING THROUGH EXPERIENCE

1. Examine your beliefs about God. Have you struggled with contradictory beliefs that have created a "dualistic" belief about God and the universe?

2. What belief can you change as a result of seeing that God is love?

3. After completing this book, consider why you do what you do in governance of yourself. Why do you avoid lying? adultery? stealing? Is it because God has a rule and if you break it he will punish you, and you don't want to get punished?

Are you afraid there are angels keeping record of all your sins and one day you will have to face judgment and get your just penalty? Or is it because you have come to understand God, his law, methods and principles, and have been won to trust? Has trust opened your heart to him and allowed you to experience transformation?

Have you come to understand that the law of love is the law of life, and breaking this law damages you, destroys God's image within you, misrepresents God and injures others? Have you come to gladly obey God because it makes so much good sense?

Glossary

Amygdala: The brain's "alarm" center and the region associated with the emotions of fear and anxiety; is involved in emotional learning and memory. Its activity is increased by stress, trauma, selfish behavior, resentment, guilt and relational conflict, and is calmed by worshiping a God of love, by engaging in meditation and altruistic behaviors, by resolving guilt and resentment, and by involvement in supportive relationships.

Anterior Cingulate Cortex (ACC): The brain region considered to be the neurological "heart." It is the seat of will (choice) and involved in empathy, altruism, sympathy, other-centered love and compassion. It is damaged by excessive limbic system activity, such as addictions, unremitting fear and anxiety, and is strengthened by meditating on God's character of love, exercising self-discipline and engaging in altruistic behaviors.

Axon: The cable-like extension from a neuronal cell body, through which the neuron sends signals.

Dendrite: The cable-like extensions from a neuronal cell body, through which the neuron receives signals.

Dorsolateral Prefrontal Cortex (DLPFC): The brain region primarily associated with reason, the ability to strategize, plan, organize, attend, mentally focus, problem-solve and provide cognitive control. It is damaged in all disorders in which the above abilities are impaired (intoxication, attention deficit hyperactivity disorder [ADHD], schizophrenia, depression, mania, Alzheimer's disease).

Glia (microglia, astroglia, oligodendricytes, Schwann cells): Brain cells that compose the white matter of the brain and provide nutritional support to keep the neurons healthy and improve signaling between neurons.

Hippocampus: The brain region associated with memory and new learning and the region that registers the rise in stress hormones and signals the hypothalamus to stop its call for more stress hormones.

Hypothalmus: The brain region that responds to the brain's emotional signals and directs the functioning of the pituitary gland.

Neuron: A "nerve" cell, composing the gray matter of the brain. Neurons are the brain cells that think, perceive and act. They communicate with electrical and chemical signals.

Orbital Prefrontal Cortex (OPFC): The brain region associated with correcting and inhibiting socially inappropriate behavior. Its activity is increased in depression and decreased in intoxication, mania and ADHD.

Pituitary Gland: The "master gland," which receives direction from the hypothalamus and sends hormone signals to the body's glands, governing their functions.

Synapse: The small gap between axons and dendrites in which chemicals pass, allowing one neuron to signal another neuron.

Thalamus: The brain's central hub for the relay of sensory and motor signals from one part of the brain to another. Its activity is essential for consciousness, is involved in sleep regulation, and contributes to a sense of what is real and what is not real.

Ventromedial Prefrontal Cortex (VMPFC): The brain region associated with moral and ethical decision making, emotional processing, empathy, and which finds meaning in life events. Its activity is decreased in depression and increased in mania.

Notes

PREFACE

[1]H. Pilcher, "The Science of Voodoo: When Mind Attacks Body," *New Scientist* (May 16-22, 2009): 30.

[2]A. M. Davis and B. H. Natelson, "Brain-Heart Interactions: The Neurocardiology of Arrhythmia and Sudden Cardiac Death," *Texas Heart Institute Journal* 20, no. 3 (1993): 158-69. W. B. Cannon, "'Voodoo' Death," *American Anthropologist* 44 (1942) (new series): 169-181. G. Engel, "Sudden and Rapid Death During Psychological Stress," *Annals of Internal Medicine* 74 (1971): 771-82. C. P. Richter, "On the Phenomenon of Sudden Death in Animal and Man," *Psychosomatic Medicine* 19 (1957): 191-98. Martin Samuels, "Contemporary Reviews in Cardiovascular Medicine: The Brain-Heart Connection," *Circulation* 116 (2007): 77-84.

[3]Pilcher, "The Science of Voodoo," p. 30. C. K. Meador, "Hex Death: Voodoo Magic or Persuasion," *Southern Medical Journal* 85 (1992): 244-67.

[4]Joel B. Green and Mark D. Baker, *Rediscovering the Scandal of the Cross* (Downers Grove, IL: InterVarsity Press, 2000), p. 28.

CHAPTER 1: GOD IS LOVE

[1]"Losing My Religion? No, Says Baylor Religion Survey," Baylor University Media Communications, September 11, 2006, www.baylor.edu/mediacommunications /news.php?action=story&story=41678.

[2]Andrew Newberg and Mark Robert Waldman, *How God Changes Your Brain: Breakthrough Findings from a Leading Neuroscientist* (New York: Random House, 2009), pp. 27-32, 53.

[3]Ibid., pp. 19-20, 36 39, 53.

[4]Stephen Post, *Altruism and Health Perspectives from Empirical Research* (New York: Oxford University Press, 2007), pp. 20-21.

[5]Ibid., p. 22.

[6]Ibid., p. 26.

CHAPTER 2: THE HUMAN BRAIN AND BROKEN LOVE

[1]IBM Systems and Technology Data Sheet at: http://public.dhe.ibm.com/common/ ssi/ecm/en/pod03034usen/POD03034USEN.PDF.

[2]A kilobyte (KB) is one thousand bytes, or single bits of information. A megabyte (MB) is 1,000 KB or one million bytes, a gigabyte (GB) is 1,000 MB or one billion bytes, and a terabyte is 1,000 GB or one trillion bytes. These measures refer to memory storage capacity or how many bits of information can be stored.

[3]"Is Watson the Smartest Machine on Earth?" Computer Science and Electrical

Engineering Department page, UMBC, Feb. 10, 2011, at www.csee.umbc
.edu/2011/02/is-watson-the-smartest-machine-on-earth/.

[4]R. Banati, "Neuropathological Imaging: *In Vivo* Detection of Glial Activation as
a Measure of Disease and Adaptive Change in the Brain," *British Medical Bulletin*
65, no. 1 (2003): 121-31. S. Herculano-Houzel and R. Lent, "Isotropic Fraction-
ator: A Simple, Rapid Method for the Quantification of Total Cell and Neuron
Numbers in the Brain," *The Journal of Neuroscience* 25, no. 10 (March 9, 2005):
2518-21.

[5]A teraflop is a measurement of processing speed; one teraflop equals one trillion
point operations per second. RAM stands for "random access memory" and basically means memory storage that can be accessed directly in any order or fashion.
This would be analogous to working memory. The more RAM the faster a computer can carry out its functions.

[6]L. Mearian, "Brain Behind IBM's Watson Not Unlike a Human's," *Computer
World*, February 18, 2011, www.computerworld.com/s/article/9210319/Brain_
behind_IBM_s_Watson_not_unlike_a_human_s.

[7]K. Jennings, "My Puny Human Brain," Slate.com, February 16, 2011, www.slate
.com/articles/arts/culturebox/2011/02/my_puny_human_brain.html.

[8]J. Sherin and C. Nemeroff, "Post-Traumatic Stress Disorder: The Neurobiological Impact of Psychological Trauma," *Dialogues in Clinical Neuroscience* 13,
no. 3 (September 2011): 263-78.

[9]L. Peoples, "Will, Anterior Cingulate Cortex, and Addiction," *Science* 296 (May
2002): 1693-94. T. Paus, "Primate Anterior Cingulate Cortex: Where Motor Control, Drive and Cognition Interface," *Neuroscience* 2 (June 2001): 418-24.

[10]T. A. Hare, C. F. Camerer and A. Rangel, "Self-Control in Decision-Making
Involves Modulation of the vmPFC Valuation System," *Science* 324, no. 5927 (May
1, 2009): 646-48. H. R. Heerkeren et al., "An fMRI Study of Simple Ethical Deci-
sion-Making," *Neuroreport* 14, no. 9 (July 2003): 1215-19. Samuel M. McClure,
David I. Laibson, George Loewenstein and Jonathan D. Cohen, "Separate Neural
Systems Value Immediate and Delayed Monetary Rewards," *Science* 306, no. 5695
(October 15, 2004): 503-7. Jorge Moll, Paul J. Eslinger and Ricardo de Oliveira-
Souza, "Frontopolar and Anterior Temporal Cortex Activation in a Moral Judg-
ment Task: Preliminary Functional MRI Results in Normal Subjects," *Arq. Neu-
ropsiquiatr.* 59, no. 3 (September 2001). Jorge Moll, Ricardo de Oliveira-Souza,
Paul J. Eslinger, Ivanei E. Bramati, Janaína Mourão-Miranda, Pedro Angelo
Andreiuolo and Luiz Pessoa, "The Neural Correlates of Moral Sensitivity: A Func-
tional Magnetic Resonance Imaging Investigation of Basic and Moral Emotions,"
The Journal of Neuroscience 22, no. 7 (April 1, 2002): 2730-36. L. Rameson et al.,
"The Neural Correlates of Empathy: Experience, Automaticity, and Prosocial
Behavior," *Journal of Cognitive Neuroscience* 24, no. 1 (January 2012): 235-45.

[11]M. Koenigs and J. Grafman, "The Functional Neuroanatomy of Depression: Distinct Roles for Ventromedial and Dorsolateral Prefrontal Cortex," *Behavioural
Brain Research* 201, no. 2 (2009): 239-43.

[12]B. Völlm et al., "Neurobiological Substrates of Antisocial and Borderline Personality Disorder: Preliminary Results of a Functional fMRI Study," *Criminal Behavioral and Mental Health* 14, no. 1 (March 2004): 39-54. L. Peoples, "Will, Anterior Cingulate Cortex, and Addiction," *Science* 296 (May 2002): 1693-94. T. R. Franklin et al., "Decreased Gray Matter Concentrations in the Insular, Orbitofrontal, Cingulate, and Temporal Cortices of Cocaine Patients," *Biological Psychiatry* 51, no. 2 (January 15, 2002): 134-42. L. van Elst, "Frontolimbic Brain Abnormalities in Patients with Borderline Personality Disorder," *Biological Psychiatry* 54, no. 2 (July 15, 2003): 163-71. J. Sherin and C. Nemeroff, "Post-Traumatic Stress Disorder: The Neurobiological Impact of Psychological Trauma," *Dialogues in Clinical Neuroscience* 13, no. 3 (September 2011): 263-78. S. Woodward and D. Kapoupek et al., "Decreased Anterior Cingulate Volume in Combat-Related PTSD," *Biological Psychiatry* 59 (2006): 582-87.

[13]N. Volkow and J. Fowler, "Addiction, a Disease of Compulsion and Drive: Involvement of the Orbitofrontal Cortex," *Cerebral Cortex* 10, no. 3 (2000): 318-25. A. Newberg, *How God Changes Your Brain* (New York: Random House, 2009), pp. 52-53.

[14]Y. Kaufman et al., "Cognitive Decline in Alzheimer Disease: Impact of Spirituality, Religiosity, and QOL," *Neurology* 68, no. 18 (May 1, 2007): 1509-14. G. Pagnoni and M. Cekic, "Age Effects on Gray Matter Volume and Attentional Performance in Zen Meditation," *Neurobiology of Aging* 28, no. 10 (October 2007): 1623-27. S. Brown et al., "Mild, Short-Term Stress Alters Dendritic Morphology in Rat Medial Prefrontal Cortex," *Cerebral Cortex* 11 (November 15, 2005): 1714-22. S. C. Cook and C. L. Wellman, "Chronic Stress Alters Dendritic Morphology in Rat Medial Prefrontal Cortex," *Journal of Neurobiology* 60, no. 2 (August 2004): 236-48. C. L. Wellman, "Dendritic Reorganization in Pyramidal Neurons in Medial Prefrontal Cortex After Chronic Corticosterone Administration," *Journal of Neurobiology* 49, no. 3 (November 15, 2001): 245-53. K. I. Pargament, H. G. Koenig, N. Tarakeshwar and J. Hahn, "Religious Struggle as a Predictor of Mortality Among Medically Ill Elderly Patients: A 2-year Longitudinal Study," *Archives of Internal Medicine* 161, no. 15 (August 13-17, 2001): 1881-85. Newberg, *How God Changes Your Brain*, p. 53. Claudia Perez-Cruz, Jeanine I. H. Müller-Keuker, Urs Heilbronner, Eberhard Fuchs and Gabriele Flügge, "Morphology of Pyramidal Neurons in the Rat Prefrontal Cortex: Lateralized Dendritic Remodeling by Chronic Stress," *Neural Plasticity* (2007), Article ID 46276. doi:10.1155/2007/46276.

CHAPTER 3: THE INFECTION OF FEAR

[1]When Scripture tells us to fear God, it is not speaking of anxiety, dread or terror, but of awe, admiration, reverence, adoration and respect. Revelation 14:7 states, "Fear God and give him glory." In other words, those who are to fear him are the ones who will be bringing him glory. These are his faithful ones, those who love him. And the Bible states that "perfect love drives out fear" (1 Jn 4:18). Therefore, those who love and glorify God won't have fear (terror, dread, anxiety) but will

have awe, admiration, adoration and respect for God.

[2]A. H. Miller et al., "Inflammation and Its Discontents: The Role of Cytokines in the Pathophysiology of Major Depression," *Biological Psychiatry* 65, no. 9 (2009): 732-41. E. Sjögren et al., "Interleukin-6 Levels in Relation to Psychosocial Factors: Studies on Serum, Daliva, and In Vitro Production by Blood Mononuclear Cells," *Brain, Behavior, and Immunity* 20, no. 3 (2006): 270-78. N. A. Harrison et al., "Inflammation Causes Mood Changes Through Alterations in Subgenual Cingulated Activity and Mesolimbic Connectivity," *Biological Psychiatry* 66, no 5 (2009): 407-14.

[3]The limbic system refers to a group of brain structures, including the amygdala, hippocampus and others, that sit above the brain stem and below the cortex. It is involved in our emotions of aggression, anger, sex drive, fear and pleasure. It also is important for new learning and memory formation.

[4]J. Medina, "The Epigenetics of Stress," *Psychiatric Times* (April 2010): 16.

[5]G. Chechik et al., "Neuronal Regulation: A Mechanism for Synaptic Pruning During Brain Maturation," *Neural Computation* 11, no. 8 (November 15, 1999): 2061-80. E. Sowell et al., "Localizing Age-Related Changes in Brain Structure Between Childhood and Adolescence Using Statistical Parametric Mapping," *Neuroimage* 9, no. 6 (June 1999): 587-97.

[6]Susan Donaldson James, ABC News brief, May 7, 2008, www.achsa.net/upload/File/Newsletters/2008/06_June/Links/6-01_Update/CW/ARTICLE%2005-07-08%20Wild%20Child%20Speechless%20After%20Tortured%20Life,%20ABC%20News,%205-7-08.pdf. J. A. Singh, "Asia and Africa: Wolf Children and Feral Man," *American Anthropologist* 45, no. 3 (July-September 1943): 468-72.

[7]Educational programming refers to media designed to engage critical thinking, memory or some other learning experience. Research has documented that children age two and younger have delayed language development from exposure to educational television in a dose-dependent fashion. The greater the exposure, the more profound the effect. This negative effect from educational television was not observed in children older than two years of age (*Journal of Pediatrics* 151, no. 4 [2007]: 364). Research such as this has led the American Academy of Pediatrics to recommend no television for children under the age of two and strict limits on older children (*Pediatrics* 107, no. 2 [February 1, 2001]: 423-26).

[8]B. Centerwall, "Television and Violence: The Scale of the Problem and Where to Go from Here," *Journal of American Medical Association* 267, no. 22 (June 10, 1992): 3059-63.

[9]F. Zimmerman and D. Christakis, "Associations Between Content Types of Early Media Exposure and Subsequent Attentional Problems," *Pediatrics* 120, no. 5 (November 5, 2007): 986-92.

[10]G. Wingwood et al., "A Prospective Study of Exposure to Rap Music Videos and African American Female Adolescents' Health," *American Journal of Public Health* 93, no. 3 (March 2003): 437-39. T. N. Robinson, H. L. Chen and J. D. Killen, "Television and Music Video Exposure and Risk of Adolescent Alcohol Use," *Pediatrics* 102, no. 50 (November 1, 1998): e54.

[11]A. Danese et al., "Adverse Childhood Experiences and Adult Risk Factors for Age-Related Disease," *Archives of Pediatrics & Adolescent Medicine* 162, no. 12 (2009): 1135-43.
[12]H. Yamasue, K. Kasai, A. Iwanami et al., "Voxel-Based Analysis of MRI Reveals Anterior Cingulate Gray-Matter Volume Reduction in Posttraumatic Stress Disorder Due to Terrorism," *Proceedings of the National Academy of Sciences of the United States of America* 100 (2003): 9039-43.
[13]Y. I. Sheline, "3D MRI Studies of Neuroanatomical Changes in Unipolar Major Depression: The Role of Stress and Medical Comorbidity," *Biological Psychiatry* 48, no. 8 (2000): 791-800. Y. K. Kim, K. Na, K. Shink et al., "Cytokine Imbalance in the Pathophysiology of Major Depressive Disorder," *Prog Neuro-Psychopharmacology & Biological Psychiatry* 31, no. 5 (2007): 1044-53. D. Musselman et al., "The Relationship of Depression to Cardiovascular Disease," *Archives of General Psychiatry* 55, no. 7 (1998): 580-92.
[14]N. Vasic, H. Walter, A. Hose and R. C. Wolf, "Gray Matter Reduction Associated with Psychopathology and Cognitive Dysfunction in Unipolar Depression: A Voxel-Based Morphometry Study," *Journal of Affective Disorders* 109, no. 1-2 (2008): 107-16. Y. I. Sheline et al., "Untreated Depression and Hippocampal Volume Loss," *American Journal of Psychiatry* 160, no. 8 (2003): 1516-18. G. Rajkowska, "Histopathology of the Prefrontal Cortex in Major Depression: What Does It Tell Us About Dysfunctional Monoaminergic Circuits?" *Progress in Brain Research* 126 (2000): 397-412. G. Rajkowska and J. J. Miguel-Hidalgo, "Gliogenesis and Glial Pathology in Depression," *CNS Neurol Disord Drug Targets* 6 (2007): 219-33. G. Rajkowska, J. J. Miguel-Hidalgo, P. Dubey, C. A. Stockmeier and K. R. Krishnan, "Prominent Reduction in Pyramidal Neurons Density in the Orbitofrontal Cortex of Elderly Depressed Patients," *Biological Psychiatry* 58 (2005): 297-306. G. Rajkowska, J. J. Miguel-Hidalgo, J. Wei, G. Dilley, S. D. Pittman, H. Y. Meltzer et al., "Morphometric Evidence for Neuronal and Glial Prefrontal Cell Pathology in Major Depression," *Biological Psychiatry* 45 (1999): 1085-98. X. Si, J. J. Miguel-Hidalgo, G. O'Dwyer, C. A. Stockmeier and G. Rajkowska, "Age-Dependent Reductions in the Level of Glial Fibrillary Acidic Protein in the Prefrontal Cortex in Major Depression," *Neuropsychopharmacology* 29 (2004): 2088-96. W. C. Drevets, "Functional Anatomical Abnormalities in Limbic and Prefrontal Cortical Structures in Major Depression," *Progress in Brain Research* 126 (2000): 413-31. D. Ongür, W. C. Drevets and J. L. Price, "Glial Reduction in the Subgenual Prefrontal Cortex in Mood Disorders," *Proceedings of the National Academy of Sciences of the United States of America* 95 (1998): 13290-95. E. Gould, "Serotonin and Hippocampal Neurogenesis," *Neuropsychopharmacology* 21 (1999): 46S-51S. S. R. Duman et al., "A Molecular and Cellular Theory of Depression," *Archives of General Psychiatry* 54, no. 7 (1997): 597-606. M. Kojima et al., "Pre and Post Synaptic Modification by Neurotrophins," *Neuroscience Research* 43, no. 3 (2002): 193-99.
[15]By terminating unhealthy relationships I do not mean that we refuse to minister to

the spiritually immature and relationally destructive. What I mean is that we do not trust the untrustworthy with our hearts, our intimacies, our plans. We don't confide in, rely on or seek support from those who will only exploit, break trust, betray and otherwise inflict injury. But we do still seek to reach them with God's love so they might experience healing of their hearts and minds.

CHAPTER 4: FREEDOM TO LOVE

[1] If you really do try this, do so with caution—and be prepared to undo the day's damage with a careful explanation.

[2] If you are the one feeling legitimate, God-given freedom infringed on, consider what you might do to start taking it back. If an honest conversation with your spouse is not possible, you might want to seek professional advice.

[3] H. K. Teng et al., "ProBDNF Induces Neuronal Apoptosis via Activation of a Receptor Complex of p75^{NTR} and Sortilin," *The Journal of Neuroscience* 25, no. 22 (June 1, 2005): 5455-63.

[4] G. Nagappan et al., "Control of Extracellular Cleavage of ProBDNF by High Frequency Neuronal Activity," *Proceedings of the National Academy of Sciences* 106, no. 4 (January 27, 2009): 1267-72.

[5] Y. Ogino et al., "Inner Experience of Pain: Imagination of Pain While Viewing Images Showing Painful Events Forms Subjective Pain Representation," *Cerebral Cortex* 17, no. 5 (2007): 1139-46. K. Herholz and Wolf-Dieter Heiss, "Functional Imaging Correlates of Recovery After Stroke in Humans," *Journal of Cerebral Blood Flow & Metabolism* 20 (2000): 1619-31. M. Lotze et al., "The Musician's Brain: Functional Imaging of Amateurs and Professionals During Performance and Imagery," *Neuroimage* 20, no. 3 (2003): 1817-29.

[6] L. Peoples, "Will, Anterior Cingulate Cortex, and Addiction," *Science* 296 (May 31, 2002): 1623.

[7] Joel Green and Mark Baker, *Rediscovering the Scandal of the Cross* (Downers Grove, IL: InterVarsity Press, 2000), p. 51.

[8] A. Newberg, *How God Changes Your Brain* (New York: Random House, 2009), p. 53.

[9] M. Milad et al., "A Role for the Human Dorsal Anterior Cingulate Cortex in Fear Expression," *Biological Psychiatry* 62, no. 10 (November 15 2007): 1191-94. P. Rudebeck et al., "Distinct Contributions of Frontal Areas to Emotion and Social Behaviour in the Rat," *European Journal of Neuroscience* 26, no. 8 (October 2007): 2315-26. A. Etkin and T. Wagner, "Emotional Processing in PTSD, Social Anxiety Disorder, and Specific Phobia," *American Journal of Psychiatry* 164, no. 10 (October 2007): 1476-88. J. Knippenberg, "N150 in Amygdalar ERPs in the Rat: Is There Modulation by Anticipatory Fear?" *Physiology & Behavior* 93, no. 1-2 (January 28, 2008): 222-28. J. Sherin and C. Nemeroff, "Post-Traumatic Stress Disorder: the Neurobiological Impact of Psychological Trauma," *Dialogues in Clinical Neuroscience* 13, no. 3 (September 2011): 263-278.

[10] R. Kanai et al., "Political Orientations Are Correlated with Brain Structure in Young Adults," *Current Biology* 21, no. 8 (April 7, 2011): 677-80.

[11]E. Maguire et al., "London Taxi Drivers and Bus Drivers: A Structural MRI and Neuropsychological Analysis," *Hippocampus* 16 (2006): 1091-1101.

[12]When God formed Adam's body out of the dirt of the earth, the body wasn't alive until God breathed into Adam the "breath" of life and Adam became a living being (Gen 2:7). The "breath" breathed into Adam is the Hebrew *neshamah*, the same "breath" of life the animals receive (Gen 7:21-22; Eccles 3:19). And when a person dies there is "no breath [*neshamah*, life] left in him" (1 Kings 17:17 KJV). But, interestingly, even though this "breath" is no longer in the dead body, Scripture uses a different word to describe what returns to God at death.

Ecclesiastes tells us that, at death, the *ruach* returns to God who gave it (Eccles 12:7). *Ruach* occurs 377 times in the Old Testament and is translated "breath" of the body thirty-three times, as in Ezekiel 37:5. So, on the surface, one could argue that God gave the "breath" of life and at death it returns to God. Yet, *ruach* is also translated as "spirit" or "strength" as in vitality seventy-six times (Judg 15:19), "courage" (Josh 2:11), "temper" (Judg 8:3), the seat of emotions three times (1 Sam 1:15), moral character sixteen times (Ezek 11:19), and the "mind" nine times (Ezek 11:5). What this suggests is that the "breath" given to Adam became personalized, and what returns to God is more than just life energy, it is the individuality of the sentient being.

Jesus said in Matthew 10:28 that we must not fear the one who destroys the body but the one who can destroy both body and soul. The Greek for soul is ψυχή (*psyche*), from where we get "psyche," which is the root for words like psychiatry and psychology, and it means the individuality or consciousness of the person. And in 1 Thessalonians chapter 4 Paul says this:

> Brothers, we do not want you to be ignorant about those who fall *asleep*, or to grieve like the rest of men, who have no hope. We believe that Jesus died and rose again and so we believe that *God will bring with Jesus those who have fallen asleep in him*. According to the Lord's own word, we tell you that we who are still alive, who are left till the coming of the Lord, *will certainly not precede those who have fallen asleep*. For the Lord himself will come down from heaven, with a loud command, with the voice of the archangel and with the trumpet call of God, and *the dead in Christ will rise first. After that*, we who are still alive and are left will be caught up together with them in the clouds to meet the Lord in the air. And so we will be with the Lord forever. (1 Thess 4:13-17, emphasis added)

Did you notice that Paul uses the same language of sleep to describe death as Jesus did? And did you notice that the concern Paul is addressing is the fear the believers had that those alive on the earth might *precede* or go to heaven before those who have fallen asleep? So, Paul says something interesting, stating that when Christ returns he will bring with him those who have fallen asleep and will resurrect them to life. Paul assures his readers that we who are alive on earth won't go to heaven until *after* our departed loved ones arise to life again. So how do we put all of this together? Let's go back to our computer analogy.

I have electronic medical records in my office. I use a laptop connected via a wireless connection to a server in another room. Everything I record on my laptop is automatically backed up on the server in the other room. If someone were to destroy my laptop, smash it, melt it, we could say that my laptop is "dead." But if I get a new piece of hardware (a new laptop) and connect it to my server and download all the stored information I have just "resurrected" my laptop.

I believe this is what Jesus and the Bible are teaching. During our lives, everything we do, all the choices we make are forming our characters, our individualities. And everything going on in the mind is recorded (backed up) perfectly in the "Lamb's book of life," God's heavenly "server." If someone kills us—"destroys the body"—they cannot touch the *psyche*—our individuality, which is stored perfectly safe in heaven. When we die, the spirit (*ruach*), our unique individuality, returns to God, safely stored awaiting download into a new body. Then when Christ returns he brings with him the stored individualities of all the saints and downloads them into perfect bodies created by Christ, and thus they are resurrected to live eternally, joining those who are alive and transformed in the twinkling of an eye. We will discuss the end of the wicked in a later chapter.

CHAPTER 7: LOVE STANDS FIRM
[1]Editors of *People Magazine*, "The Killer and the Kids," *People: Amazing Stories of Survival* (New York: Time Life, Inc., 2006), p. 107.

CHAPTER 8: CHANGING OUR VIEW OF GOD
[1]I recommend the book *Genetic Entropy and the Mystery of the Genome* by Dr. John C. Sanford, an applied geneticist at Cornell University. He describes with sound scientific evidence how the human genome has degraded and continues to degrade since sin. He also describes how natural selection cannot select out the multitude of new mutations that occur with each generation. Such genetic mutations, accumulating with each generation, document one way in which God's creation is damaged and weighed down by sin.

CHAPTER 9: THE POWER OF TRUTH
[1]A. Newberg, *How God Changes Your Brain* (New York: Random House, 2009), p. 49.

CHAPTER 11: ENLARGING OUR VIEW OF GOD
[1]Tragic events, pain and suffering happen in this world for a variety of reasons, and not everyone undergoing such difficulties are in the position of Job or Harold. This story serves only to highlight one reason among many why, in some circumstances, God allows suffering.
[2]Some may recall that when Christ performed miracles he often said, "Your faith has made you well" (Mk 5:34 GNT) and be concerned that my position in this chapter is selective and skewed. Miracles happened in the lives of individuals as they exercised trust or faith in God/Christ. Faith was the opening of the heart to allow God's power to work in them. So Christ's statement is understood to mean

that only with faith was God able to work in the person's life to bring healing. But when weighed against the evidence throughout the rest of Scripture, it would be erroneous to conclude that Christ's statement indicates that such faith is strong or mature faith. In fact, the evidence from the narrative would suggest the vast majority of those whose faith made them well were new to faith, and the miracles were beneficial in solidifying that faith. So the point remains: miracles are often through the strong in faith for the benefit of the weak in faith, and failure to experience a miracle is not, in itself, evidence of a lack of faith.

CHAPTER 12: THE JUDGEMENT OF GOD

[1]A. H. Miller et al., "Inflammation and Its Discontents: The Role of Cytokines in the Pathophysiology of Major Depression," *Biological Psychiatry* 65, no. 9 (2009): 732-41. S. Alesci et al., "Major Depression Is Associated with Significant Diurnal Elevations in Plasma Interleukin-6 Levels, a Shift of Its Circadian Rhythm, and Loss of Physiological Complexity in Its Secretion: Clinical Implications," *Journal of Clinical Endocrinology & Metabolism* 90, no. 5 (2005): 2522-30. V. Vaccarino et al., "Depressive Symptoms and Risk of Functional Decline and Death in Patients with Heart Failure," *Journal of the American College of Cardiology* 38 (2001): 199-205. S. A. Everson et al., "Depressive Symptoms and Increased Risk of Stroke Mortality Over a 29-Year Period," *Archives of Internal Medicine* 158 (1998): 1133-38. W. W. Eaton et al., "The Influence of Educational Attainment on Depression and Risk of Type 2 Diabetes," *Diabetes Care* 19, no. 10 (1996): 1097-1102. R. Coelho et al., "Bone Mineral Density and Depression: A Community Study of Women," *Journal of Psychosomatic Research* 46 (1999): 29-35. D. Michelson et al., "Depression and Osteoporosis: Epidemiology and Potential Mediating Pathways," *New England Journal of Medicine* 335 (1996): 1176-81. A. E. Yazici et al., "Bone Mineral Density in Premenopausal Women with Major Depression," *Joint Bone Spine* 72 (2005): 540-43.

CHAPTER 13: IN THE BRAIN OF CHRIST

[1]D. Grogan, "'To Save Their Daughter From Leukemia, Abe and Mary Ayala Conceived a Plan—and a Baby," *People Magazine* 33, no. 9 (March 5, 1990): www.people.com/people/archive/article/0,,20116976,00.html.

[2]M. Inbar, "Born to Save Sister's Life, She's 'Glad I Am in This Family,'" *Today.com* (June 3, 2011): http://today.msnbc.msn.com/id/43265160/ns/today-good_news/t/born-save-sisters-life-shes-glad-i-am-family/.

[3]Jim McHugh, "Born to Save a Life," *People: Amazing Stories of Survival* (New York: Time Inc., 2006), p. 115.

[4]W. Kaiser et al., *Hard Sayings of the Bible* (Downers Grove, IL: InterVarsity Press, 1996), pp. 542-43.

[5]James K. Beilby and Paul R. Eddy, *The Nature of the Atonement* (Downers Grove, IL: InterVarsity Press, 2006).

[6]Robert S. Franks, *A History of the Doctrine of the Work of Christ in Its Ecclesiastical Development*, vol. 1 (London: Hodder and Stoughton, 1918), p. 21.

[7]Ibid., p. 22.

[8]Ibid., pp. 37-38.

[9]Beilby and Eddy, *Nature of the Atonement*, p. 137.

[10]The point here is not to argue for or against any specific change to the Decalogue. I simply use this asserted change in the Commandments as evidence that Christianity has accepted an imposed law-construct. For if the law was still viewed as natural, like gravity or respiration, would any Christian group think they could change it? "The church after changing the day of rest from the Jewish Sabbath or seventh-day of the week to the first, made the third commandment refer to Sunday as the day to be kept holy as the Lord's day," *Catholic Encyclopedia*, vol. 4, p. 153.

[11]Peter Leithart, *Defending Constantine* (Downers Grove, IL: IVP Academic, 2010), pp. 302-3.

[12]T. Jennings, *Could It Be This Simple?* (Hagerstown, MD: Autumn House, 2007), pp. 101-2.

[13]The paraphrase of Romans 7 found at the end of chapter 5 demonstrates the application of this concept.

[14]Kaiser et al., *Hard Sayings of the Bible*, pp. 542-43.

[15]O. Heinrich, "A Hollowed Spot," *Southern Tidings* 63, no. 10 (October 1969): 12-13. See also www.adventistcamps.org/article/80/camp-directory/cohutta-springs-youth -camp.

[16]"Atone: short for the phrase 'set or make at one' . . . make one, put at one, unite . . . From the frequent phrases 'set at one' or 'at onement,' the combined *atonement* began to take the place of *onement* early in the sixteenth century; and *atone* to supplant *one* as the verb form around 1550. *Atone* was not admitted into the Bible until 1611, though *atonement* had been in since William Tyndale." From J. Simpson and S. Weiner, *The Oxford English Dictionary*, 2nd ed. (Oxford: Clarendon Press, 1989), pp. 754-55.

[17]C. Thomspon, *Anatomy of the Soul* (Carol Stream, IL: Tyndale House, 2010), p. 170.

[18]The Bible uses many metaphors to describe Jesus' work in our salvation, or atonement. However, behind the metaphors exist a reality, a cosmologic truth on which this universe runs. It is the position of this book that this truth is God's character of love. And that character of love is expressed in the law of love, the template on which life is constructed to operate. If this is true, then all metaphors will find their truest meaning in this reality. I would like to demonstrate how this *could* be a unifying perspective:

Ransom Metaphor: Jesus said he would give his life as a ransom for many. A ransom is the price necessary in order to free someone held in captivity or bondage. What holds us in bondage? The lies we believe about God and our own fallen nature. Then what would be the price to set us free? The truth about God, which destroys lies and restores trust, and a new nature. Jesus Christ provided these through his earthly ministry. Thus the ransom price is paid to us, because the reality of our condition requires it. It would be analogous to a renal failure patient receiving a kidney. The one donating the kidney is "paying a high price" and even "ransoming" the patient from captivity in renal failure by paying the price necessary to free them from that terminal condition. And to whom is the kidney "paid"? The one who is dying. Why? Because their condition requires it in order to be put back in harmony with the way life was built to operate.

The Moral Influence Theory would promote the first half of this ransom price; namely, the truth about God revealed in Christ, which wins us to trust. In that trust relationship, God does the rest to heal and restore the sinner back into harmony with the law of love, as long as the sinner follows God's direction. The moral influence theory leaves undeveloped the other elements of Christ's work.

Christus Victor Model, or defeating Satan and his power. We must first identify the source of Satan's power, which arises in two ways: the power of lies as described in chapter 2; and secondarily, the power of God's violated law. Why does holding someone's head under water destroy them? Because the law of respiration is noncompromising, and to violate it exerts a destructive power that humanity cannot overcome. Likewise, God's law of love, or the design for life, is noncompromising and to violate it exerts a destructive power humanity cannot overcome. The only way to overcome being held under water is to get an air source. The only way to overcome Satan's power is to receive the truth to destroy lies, and connect to a source of perfect love.

Christ's death destroyed "him who holds *the power of death*—that is, the devil" (Heb 2:14, emphasis mine). But what is the devil's power of death? If we believe death is the opposite of eternal life, then we get a significant clue in John 17:3 where Jesus stated life eternal is knowing God and his Son. If life eternal is knowing God, then death, being the opposite of life, would be not knowing God. So Satan's power of death would be the lies he tells about God, who we believe, that keep us from knowing God. Just as we discussed in chapter 2, lies believed break the circle of love and trust, and broken love and trust result in ruin and death.

Therefore, Christ achieves victory over Satan by revealing the truth about God, about himself, about the nature and character of sin, and about the devil, which disarms the devil, making his weapons of deceit useless. This is described with graphic imagery in Revelation when the rider on a white horse, whose name is the Word of God, destroys his enemies with a sword coming out of his mouth (Rev 19:11-21). Would not that sword be the sword of truth (Eph 6:17), the spoken word coming from the Word of God? What other than truth would be coming from the mouth of Jesus? And further, Christ, in his humanity, exercised his human brain to restore God's law to humanity, thereby defeating Satan's work of attempting to obliterate the image of God in humankind. I find any suggestion of a battle of power, might or physical force between Christ and Satan to be without merit, because the Creator could as easily destroy Satan as a child casts a penny to the ground. Every time Jesus confronted a demon he exercised absolute authority over them, notably before his death and resurrection.

What I have described in this note is incomplete and merely a small example of how God's character of love is the unifying center of reality. I hope others will pick up this thread and further develop the connections between God's redeeming work and his character and methods of love.

CHAPTER 14: FORGIVENESS

[1]G. W. Bush, speech to joint houses of Congress, September, 20, 2001, quoted from www.historyplace.com/speeches/gw-bush-9-11.htm.

[2]A. F. Shariff and M. Rhemtulla, "Divergent Effects of Beliefs in Heaven and Hell on National Crime Rates," PloS ONE 7, no. 6 (2012): e39048. doi:10.1371/journal.pone.0039048

[3]M. Ghandi, quoted at www.famousquotesabout.com/quote/An-eye-for-an/375503.

[4]Some are concerned that extending forgiveness to a person who refuses to repent would leave one open for repeated exploitation and injury. This concern occurs when one mistakes forgiveness for restored trust. Forgiving a person does not change the character of the offender but removes resentment and bitterness from the heart of the offended. Only when the offender repents and experiences God's transformation of the heart, such that they love others more than themselves, would it be safe to trust. So we forgive, but we base our trust on the trustworthiness of the other person.

CHAPTER 15: WHEN GOOD PREVAILS

[1]Associated Press, "Amish Girl Asked to Be Shot First to Save Classmates," Saturday, October 7, 2006.

[2]WorldNetDaily, "Grieving Amish Raise Money for Killer's Family: 'This Is Possible if You Have Christ in Your Heart,'" October 4, 2006, www.wnd.com/2006/10/38231/.

[3]J. Howell, "Gator Girl to the Rescue," People: Amazing Stories of Survival (New York: Time Inc., 2006), p. 23.

CHAPTER 16: WHEN LOVE BURNS FREE

[1]Joel Green and Mark Baker, Rediscovering the Scandal of the Cross (Downers Grove, IL: InterVarsity Press, 2000), p. 29.

[2]The Doctrine Commission of the Church of England, The Mystery of Salvation: The Story of God's Gift: A Report (London: Church House Publishing, 1995), p. 197.

[3]In a note in chapter 4, we explored what happens to the individuality of the righteous at "death," using an analogy of a computer and its server, but we left until now what happens to the wicked. The wicked will be resurrected at the end of the thousand years at the resurrection of damnation into imperfect bodies (Rev 20:5). At that time they have their individualities downloaded from God's record books (heavenly servers), and the heavenly server is "erased." No individuality is backed up or stored any longer. The New Jerusalem is on earth and a period of time goes by as the wicked gather together to attack the city (Rev 20:7-9). During this time, the righteous are in the city and the gates of the city are open (Rev 21:25). When the wicked march on the city en masse to attack it, then God unveils his full glory and the fire of his presence, the fire of truth and love, and consumes all sin as described above. What is the point of this resurrection? To reveal that God, when he put people to sleep in Old Testament times, in no way determined the ultimate outcome of their lives. The

wicked are raised to finish their lives by the exercise of their own choices. But, even with the New Jerusalem on earth, the minds of the wicked are so settled into the lies about God that they still won't surrender to him and come into the city. Thus it is proved beyond all doubt that it is unremedied sin that destroys, and God is truly the God of love and life. God stands exonerated of all charges in the minds of his intelligent creatures. The last lie, that God is the source of death, is fully disproved.

Then, when the wicked are destroyed, because their individualities are no longer stored in heaven, they are eternally annihilated, or gone. This is the death of sin, the wages of sin, eternal nonexistence. While both righteous and wicked "sleep" until resurrection, only the unhealed wicked are eternally destroyed (or die). Why? Because life was built to exist only in harmony with God's character of love; the wicked having never been restored to God's design for life cannot survive. God, in harmony with his law of love and liberty, sets them free to experience what they have chosen—eternal separation from him, the source of life—and thus they pass permanently from existence.

One premise that underlies a belief in the eternal suffering of the wicked is the idea that at creation, in Eden, God created human beings with some aspect of their being that is immortal. If true, then once rebellion occurred God's hands were tied for those who reject his mercy—they would live forever shut out from his presence and thus to suffer eternally. And as much as God would love to prevent them from suffering eternally, having already given them immortality, there is simply nothing he can do to prevent it.

I assert the idea of human beings possessing inherent immortality to be a false premise. I assert that only God is immortal (Job 4:17; Ps 6:15; 1 Tim 6:16; Rom 2:7; 1 Cor 15:51-54), and eternal life is a gift from God to human beings (Jn 3:16; Rom 6:23), who have been restored to trust and have had the law of love written within (Heb 8:10). Based on our understanding of the law of love being the design template for life, based on harmony with Scripture (like those noted in this paragraph), and believing in God's foreknowledge and sovereignty, I reject the premise that humanity possesses some aspect of inherent immortality. I find it unbelievable to think God would be foolish enough to create beings with inherent immortality, knowing they would rebel and then suffer for all eternity. Such a being would be either a cruel sadist or naive fool. God is neither. He is infinite in love, mercy and wisdom. Therefore, the position described in this chapter is one that harmonizes all three threads of evidence and confirms God as a being of love.

CHAPTER 17: BUDDHA, JESUS AND PREPARING YOUR BRAIN FOR ETERNITY

[1]P. M. Barnes, B. Bloom and R. Nahin, "Complementary and Alternative Medicine Use Among Adults and Children: United States, 2007," *National Health Statistics Reports*, no. 12 (December 10, 2008): 1-23.

[2]M. B. Ospina, T. K. Bond, M. Karkhaneh et al., "Meditation Practices for Health, State of the Research," *Evidence Report/Technology Assessment*, no. 155 (2007). S. R.

Bishop, M. Lau, S. Shapiro et al., "Mindfulness: A Proposed Operational Definition," *Clinical Psychology: Science and Practice* 11, no. 3 (2004): 230-41. P. Grossman, L. Niemann and S. Schmidt et al., "Mindfulness-Based Stress Reduction and Health Benefits: A Meta-analysis," *Journal of Psychosomatic Research* 57, no. 1 (2004): 35-43. J. K. Zinn, A. O. Massion, and J. Kristeller, "Effectiveness of a Meditation-Based Stress Reduction Program in the Treatment of Anxiety Disorders," *American Journal of Psychiatry* 149 (1992): 936-43. T. Toneatto and L. Nguyen, "Does Mindfulness Meditation Improve Anxiety and Mood Symptoms? A Review of the Controlled Research," *Canadian Journal of Psychiatry* 52, no. 4 (2007): 260-66. S. G. Hofmann, A. T. Sawyer, A. A. Witt and D. Oh, "The Effect of Mindfulness-Based Therapy on Anxiety and Depression: A Meta-analytic Review," *Journal of Consulting and Clinical Psychology* 78 (2010): 169-83. A. K. Niazi and S. K. Niazi, "Mindfulness-Based Stress Reduction, a Non-Pharmacological Approach for Chronic Illness," *North American Journal of Medical Sciences* 3 (2010): 20-23. E. Bohlmeijer, R. Prenger and E. Taal, "The Effects of Mindfulness-Based Stress Reduction Therapy on Mental Health of Adults with a Chronic Medical Disease, A Meta-analysis," *Journal of Psychosomatic Research* 68, no. 6 (2010): 539-44. J. Vollestad, B. Sivertsen and G. H. Nielsen, "Mindfulness-Based Stress Reduction for Patients with Anxiety Disorders: Evaluation in a Randomized Controlled Trial," *Behaviour Research and Therapy* 49 (2011): 281-88. T. Barnhofer, C. Crane and E. Hargus, "Mindfulness-Based Cognitive Therapy as a Treatment for Chronic Depression, a Preliminary Study," *Behaviour Research and Therapy* 47 (2009): 366-73. J. D. Teasdale, Z. V. Segal and J. M. Williams, "Prevention of Relapse/Recurrence in Major Depression by Mindfulness-Based Cognitive Therapy," *Journal of Consulting and Clinical Psychology* 68 (2000): 615-23. K. Pilkington, G. Kirkwood, H. Rampes and J. Richardson, "Yoga for Depression: The Research Evidence," *Journal of Affective Disorders* 89 (2005): 13-24. S. S. Khumar, P. Kaur and S. Kaur, "Effectiveness of Shavasana on Depression Among University Students," *Indian Journal of Clinical Psychology* 20 (199): 82-87. L. A. Uebelacker, G. Tremont, G. Epstein-Lubow et al., "Open Trial of Vinyasa Yoga for Persistently Depressed Individuals: Evidence of Feasibility and Acceptability," *Behavior Modification* 34, no. 3 (2012): 247-64. L. D. Butler, L. C. Waelde, T. A. Hastings et al., "Meditation with Yoga, Group Therapy with Hypnosis, and Psychoeducation for Long-Term Depressed Mood: A Randomized Pilot Trial," *Journal of Clinical Psychology* 64, no. 7 (2008): 806-20. N. Janakiramaiah, B. N. Gangadhar, P. J. Naga Venkatesha Murthy, M. G. Harish, D. K. Subbakrishna and A. Vedamurthachar, "Antidepressant Efficacy of Sudarshan Kriya Yoga (SKY) in Melancholia: A Randomized Comparison with Electroconvulsive Therapy (ECT) and Imipramine," *Journal of Affective Disorders* 57, no. 1-3 (2000): 255-59. A. Woolery, H. Myers, B. Sternlieb and L. Zeltzer, "A Yoga Intervention for Young Adults with Elevated Symptoms of Depression," *Alternative Therapies in Health and Medicine* 10, no. 2 (2004): 60-63. T. Kamei, Y. Toriumi, H. Kimura, S. Ohno, H. Kumano and K. Kimura, "Decrease in Serum Cortisol During Yoga Exercise Is Correlated with α Wave Activation," *Per-*

ceptual & Motor Skills 90, no. 3, part 1 (2000): 1027-32. A. Michalsen, P. Grossman, A. Acil et al., "Rapid Stress Reduction and Anxiolysis Among Distressed Women as a Consequence of a Three-Month Intensive Yoga Programme," *Medical Science Monitor* 11, no. 12 (2005): 555-61. M. R. Rao, N. Raghuram, H. R. Nagendra et al., "Anxiolytic Effects of a Yoga Program in Early Breast Cancer Patients Undergoing Conventional Treatment: A Randomized Controlled Trial," *Complementary Therapies in Medicine* 17 (2009): 1-8. G. Kirkwood, H. Rampes, V. Tuffrey, J. Richardson and K. Pilkington, "Yoga for Anxiety: A Systematic Review of the Research Evidence," *British Journal of Sports Medicine* 39, no. 12 (2005): 884-91. D. S. Shannahoff-Khalsa, L. E. Ray, S. Levine, C. C. Gallen, B. J. Schwartz and J. J. Sidorowich, "Randomized Controlled Trial of Yogic Meditation Techniques for Patients with Obsessive-Compulsive Disorder," *CNS Spectrums* 4, no. 12 (1999): 34-47. N. Gupta, S. Khera, R. P. Vempati, R. Sharma and R. L. Bijlani, "Effect of Yoga Based Lifestyle Intervention on State and Trait Anxiety," *Indian Journal of Physiology and Pharmacology* 50, no. 1 (2006): 41-47. T. Field, "Yoga Clinical Research Review," *Complementary Therapies in Clinical Practice* 17, no. 1 (2010): 1-8.

[3]J. Malan, "Eastern Meditation Sneaks into the Church," *For the Love of His Truth* blog at http://fortheloveofhistruth.com/2012/02/13/eastern-meditation-sneaks-into -the-church/.

[4]F. Klin, online report at www.scribd.com/doc/49912205/Ancient-Thought-In Modern-Dress-Spiritual-Formation-the-Seventh Day-Adventist-Church.

[5]Herbert Benson, *Timeless Healing* (New York: Scribner, 1996). A. Newberg, *How God Changes Your Brain* (New York: Random House, 2009), p. 31.

[6]Newberg, *How God Changes Your Brain*, p. 34.

[7]A. Govinda, *Foundations of Tibetan Mysticism* (London: Rider, 1969), pp. 107-8.

[8]"God Encounter" here refers to those practices within Christianity that utilize Eastern meditation techniques to achieve an altered mental and emotional state.

[9]J. Taylor, online video lecture at www.ted.com/talks/lang/en/jill_bolte_taylor _s_powerful_stroke_of_insight.html.

[10]R. Cahn and J. Polich, "Meditation States and Traits: EEG, ERP, and Neuroimaging Studies," *Psychological Bulletin* 132, no. 2 (March 2006): 180-211. Newberg, *How God Changes Your Brain*, p. 55. T. Kjaer et al., "Increased Dopamine Tone During Meditation-Induced Change of Consciousness," *Cognitive Brain Research* 13, no. 2 (April 2002): 255-59.

[11]B. Miller, "Matters of the Mind: A Look into the Psychology of Meditation," *The Daily Mind*, www.thedailymind.com/meditation/matters-of-the mind-a-look-into-the-psychology-of-meditation/.

[12]C. Thompson, *Anatomy of the Soul* (Carol Stream, IL: Tyndale House, 2010), p. 41.

[13]Ibid., pp. 34-38.

[14]Newberg, *How God Changes Your Brain*, pp. 54-55.

If you have questions or comments, would like
to share what this book has meant to you,
or if you would like a further exploration
of this topic, please visit our website
at www.ComeAndReason.com.